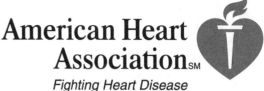

American Heart Association℠

*Fighting Heart Disease
and Stroke*

Textbook of
Basic Life Support for
Healthcare
Providers

Editors

Nisha Chibber Chandra, MD
Mary Fran Hazinski, MSN, RN

Subcommittee on Basic Life Support, 1991-1994

Nisha Chibber Chandra, MD, Chair
Loring S. Flint, MD, Immediate Past Chair
Thomas P. Aufderheide, MD
Thomas A. Barnes, EdD, RRT
Carol Belmont, RN
Elaine Keiss Daily, MSN, RN

Mary Fran Hazinski, MSN, RN
Larry W. Heinz
Richard L. Judd, PhD
Richard J. Melker, MD, PhD
William H. Montgomery, MD
James T. Niemann, MD

James L. Paturas, EMT-P
James S. Seidel, MD, PhD
Edward Stapleton, EMT-P
Samuel J. Stratton, MD

Subcommittee on Pediatric Resuscitation, 1991-1994

Mary Fran Hazinski, MSN, RN, Cochair
Linda Quan, MD, Cochair
Leon Chameides, MD, Cochair,
    1991-1993
James S. Seidel, MD, PhD, Chair,
    1987-1991
David J. Burchfield, MD

Arthur Cooper, MD
Charles J. Coté, MD
J. Michael Dean, MD
Mary E. Fallat, MD
Wayne H. Franklin, MD
Mark G. Goetting, MD
Harriet Hawkins, RNC, CCRN

Karin A. McCloskey, MD
Lyle F. McGonigle, MD
Olga E. Mohan, MD
Vinay Nadkarni, MD
John R. Raye, MD
Kathryn A. Taubert, PhD
Timothy S. Yeh, MD

Committee on Emergency Cardiac Care, 1991-1994

Joseph P. Ornato, MD, Chair
Richard E. Kerber, MD, Immediate Past
    Chair
Richard O. Cummins, MD, MPH, MSc,
    Vice Chair

Richard K. Albert, MD
Donald D. Brown, MD
Nisha Chibber Chandra, MD
Mary Fran Hazinski, MSN, RN

Richard J. Melker, MD, PhD
Linda Quan, MD
W. Douglas Weaver, MD

Reviewers

Frank X. Doto, MS
Valerie Sloboda-Mague, RN

©1994, American Heart Association

ISBN 0-87493-615-2

Contents

9 Automated External Defibrillation

Preface

This manual is provided as a textbook and reference for the American Heart Association's course in basic life support for healthcare providers. Healthcare providers include physicians, nurses, EMTs, and allied health personnel.

The manual incorporates recommendations of the 1992 National Conference on Cardiopulmonary Resuscitation (CPR) and Emergency Cardiac Care (ECC). These recommendations were published as "Guidelines for Cardiopulmonary Resuscitation and Emergency Cardiac Care" in *The Journal of the American Medical Association* in October 1992 (*JAMA.* 1992;268:2171-2302). Reprints of the "Guidelines" are available from the American Heart Association. The proceedings of the 1992 conference, which review the science that led to the formulation of the guidelines, were published in *Annals of Emergency Medicine* in February 1993.

Besides incorporating the most recent recommendations on CPR and ECC, this manual differs from the previous edition in several ways. Chapter 1 has been extensively revised to include more information about the chain of survival concept and ways to improve the total ECC system. Information about mass training and the AHA training network has been moved to the *Instructor's Manual for Basic Life Support.* Because the historical background of CPR, including the recommendations of the previous national conferences, is readily available in the "Guidelines," that material is no longer included here.

Risk factors for heart disease and prudent heart living, formerly included in chapter 2 on cardiopulmonary physiology and dysfunction, are now presented as a separate chapter to emphasize their importance. The five chapters that previously comprised adult CPR have been consolidated into a single chapter, and the section on two-rescuer CPR has been considerably simplified.

New material on the early diagnosis and management of stroke has been added because of the magnitude of this problem and because of the importance of proper early diagnosis and treatment. Additional material is provided on other special resuscitation situations, including hypothermia, electric shock and lightning strike, and cardiac arrest associated with trauma.

Chapter 6 on pediatric BLS has been extensively revised. Material has been added on the recovery position, barrier devices, and BLS in trauma, and discussions of injury prevention and other topics have been expanded and clarified.

The appendix on medicolegal considerations and decision making in CPR has been rewritten and now stands as a separate chapter on ethics and legal considerations.

Finally, a chapter on automated external defibrillators has been added to support the growing interest in defibrillation as a basic life support skill. Clinical data establish that defibrillation is the definitive therapy for many cardiac arrests. The dissemination of the skill of defibrillation supported by this chapter recognizes this fact and encourages implementation of programs in early defibrillation. Although this module is currently optional in AHA healthcare provider programs, it is highly recommended and is likely to become mandatory.

The aim throughout has been to streamline the manual so that it better meets the needs of healthcare professionals. As always, we welcome your comments and suggestions.

Basic Life Support in Perspective

This manual is designed to meet the needs of healthcare professionals who respond to cardiac and respiratory emergencies. It teaches

- The role of the healthcare provider and the community in the total emergency cardiac care (ECC) system
- The information and techniques needed for adult and pediatric cardiopulmonary resuscitation (CPR) and special rescue situations
- The anatomy and physiology of the cardiovascular and respiratory systems
- Risk factors for heart disease and stroke and the concept of prudent heart living
- Signals and actions for survival that victims and healthcare providers must take to lessen the chance of disability and to prevent sudden death
- Injury prevention in the pediatric age group
- Safety factors in training and actual rescue
- Ethical and legal considerations in CPR

Chapter 1 discusses the lifesaving potential of basic life support (BLS) and advanced cardiac life support (ACLS), explains the importance of a communitywide emergency medical service (EMS) system, and defines the role of BLS and ACLS in ECC. This chapter also presents the structural components of a "chain of survival" required to save victims of cardiac arrest.

The Need for Medical Intervention

Cardiovascular disease accounts for nearly 1 million deaths each year in the United States. Half of these deaths are due to coronary heart disease, and most of them occur suddenly.[1] It is estimated that 6.3 million Americans have significant coronary heart disease, and many of them are at risk for sudden death or myocardial infarction (Fig 1).

Although death rates from coronary heart disease and stroke have declined more than 30% since 1979 (Fig 2),[2,3] due at least in part to advances in medical treatment and healthier lifestyles, many preventable deaths still occur. Approximately two thirds of sudden deaths due to coronary heart disease occur out of the hospital, and most occur within 2 hours of the onset of cardiovascular symptoms.[2,4-9] Many of these deaths

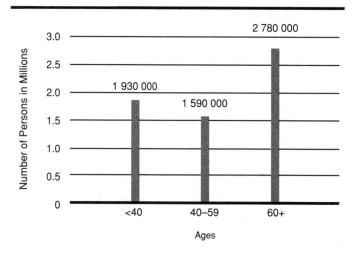

United States: 1991 Estimate

Source: National Health and Nutrition Examination Survey 1976–80, (NHANES II), National Center for Health Statistics and the American Heart Association.

Fig 1. Estimated prevalence of coronary heart disease by age.

can be prevented by prompt BLS and ACLS, including rapid access to the EMS system, bystander CPR, and early defibrillation.[10-15]

The need for these interventions is not limited to adults with coronary heart disease. Many victims of trauma, drowning, electrocution, suffocation, airway obstruction, drug intoxication, and the like may be saved by prompt initiation of such intervention. Respiratory failure, congenital anomalies, or perinatal asphyxia may result in the need for resuscitation at birth. Trauma, a leading cause of death and disability in children and young adults,[16-18] requires prompt intervention with BLS and advanced life support not only to save lives but also to help avoid devastating brain damage that results in long-term suffering and economic hardship.

The Ultimate Coronary Care Unit

Public education and training are crucial to the effort to reduce sudden death. Since the majority of sudden deaths caused by cardiac arrest occur before hospitalization, it is clear that the community must be

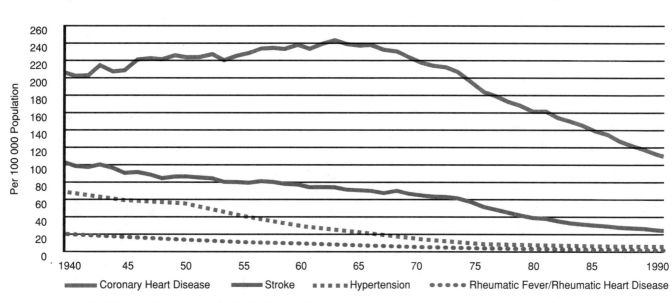

Age-adjusted to 1940 U.S. population and to the 6th Revision ICDA.
Source: National Center for Health Statistics and the American Heart Association.

Fig 2. Age-adjusted death rates for major cardiovascular diseases.

recognized as "the ultimate coronary care unit."[19]

The CPR-ECC programs described in this chapter have been and will continue to be valuable formats for educating the community about its responsibility.

Optimally the focus should be on both lifesaving techniques and prevention through reduction of risk factors.

Community training programs should incorporate education in *primary prevention,* which includes risk factor detection and modification and awareness of the signals of impending cardiovascular events, and *secondary prevention,* which is aimed at preventing sudden cardiac death and myocardial infarction in patients known to have coronary heart disease. It is clear that coronary heart disease and other forms of atherosclerotic vascular disease are supported by community nutritional patterns, prosmoking messages delivered to children, and cultural and social pressures that mold unhealthy behaviors and lifestyles.

Training nonmedical personnel in CPR saves lives that might otherwise be lost due to cardiac arrest. Communities that have high numbers of laypersons trained in lifesaving techniques such as CPR, along with a rapid response system of well-trained para-medical personnel providing ACLS, successfully resuscitate more than 40% of patients with docu-mented out-of-hospital ventricular fibrillation (a chaotic, uncoordinated quivering of the heart muscle).[20]

While the terms *BLS* and *CPR* often are used inter-changeably, it should be noted that CPR is a compo-nent of ECC that may be required in ACLS as well as in BLS.

Emergency Cardiac Care

ECC includes all responses necessary to deal with sudden and often life-threatening events affecting the cardiovascular and pulmonary systems, as well as the ultimate viability of the full-functioning human being. Cardiac disease is by far the most frequent cause of these potentially catastrophic events.

In relation to cardiac disease, ECC specifically includes

- Recognizing early warning signs of heart attack and activating the EMS system, efforts to prevent complications, reassurance of the victim, and prompt availability of monitoring equipment
- Providing immediate BLS at the scene, when needed
- Providing ACLS at the scene as quickly as pos-sible to defibrillate, if necessary, and stabilize the victim before transportation
- Transferring the stabilized victim to an appropriate hospital where definitive cardiac care can be provided

The term *emergency cardiac care* in this context extends to the care of other life-threatening catastrophic events that may not initially involve the heart, such as previously mentioned syndromes involving an obstructed airway, stroke, near-drowning, electrocution, trauma, and hypothermia. Pediatric and neonatal resuscitation are also included, even though in most instances in this age group the primary event does not occur in the heart.

Emergency transportation alone, without life support, does not constitute ECC. Although transportation is an important aspect of ECC, the major emphasis is on early provision of definitive care when needed (eg, defibrillation), use of CPR when needed, and stabilization of the victim of the life-threatening emergency (eg, control of hemorrhage). Inordinate delays at the scene must be avoided, but defibrillation when necessary and stabilization to the extent possible should be achieved before and during transport of the victim to the site of continuing care.

The two components of ECC are BLS and ACLS. CPR is an integral part of the lifesaving process in both.

CPR includes a series of assessments and interventions that support cardiac and respiratory function. If CPR is performed correctly, (1) cardiac arrest may be prevented, (2) cardiorespiratory function may be restored, or (3) cardiorespiratory function may be maintained until advanced life support is provided. CPR requires no special equipment and can be quickly mastered. Since CPR skills may be lifesaving, they should be taught to all who are capable of learning them.

Prompt bystander CPR is crucial to these resuscitative efforts.[21] In the absence of prompt bystander CPR, successful resuscitation of the out-of-hospital cardiac arrest victim is unlikely, despite the availability of a well-trained paramedical team with a rapid response time.[21]

Each person trained in CPR should have a well-formulated plan of action for use in emergency, based on local community resources and the EMS system. When symptoms occur that suggest a profound circulatory collapse and imminent cardiac arrest, a mobile life support unit should be summoned to reduce elapsed time from onset of symptoms to entry into an EMS system. In the absence of such a system, the victim should be brought without delay to an emergency department or other facility with 24-hour life support capability.

BLS is the phase of ECC that is intended

• To prevent arrested or inadequate circulation or respiration through prompt recognition and intervention, early entry into the EMS system, or both

• To support the circulation and respiration of a victim of arrest through CPR

BLS should be initiated by any person present when cardiac or respiratory arrest occurs. To be successful, ECC depends on the layperson's understanding of the importance of early activation of the EMS system and willingness and ability to initiate prompt, effective CPR. Accordingly, providing lifesaving BLS at this level can be considered primarily a public, community responsibility. The healthcare community, however, has the responsibility to provide leadership in educating the public and to support community education and training.

ACLS includes BLS plus the use of adjunctive equipment in supporting ventilation, the establishment of intravenous access, the administration of drugs, cardiac monitoring, defibrillation or other control of arrhythmias, and care after resuscitation. It also includes the establishment of communication necessary to ensure continued care. A physician must supervise and direct ACLS efforts in one of three ways: (1) in person at the scene, (2) by direct communication, or (3) by a previously defined alternative mechanism such as standing orders.

ECC should be an integral part of a total communitywide emergency medical care system. Each system should be based on local community needs for patient care and available resources and be consistent with regional, state, and national guidelines. The success of such a system requires multijurisdictional participation and planning to ensure operational and equipment compatibility within the system and between adjacent systems. The community must be willing both to fund the program it develops and to review its efficacy. The initial planning of a system should be through a local advisory council on emergency services charged with assessing community needs, defining priorities, and arranging to meet needs with available resources. Critical evaluation of operating policies, procedures, statistics, and case reports must be the continuing responsibility of the medical director. Operational activities must be evaluated against adopted protocols. Evaluation of skills of trained personnel, whether based in or out of the hospital, must be conducted on a regular schedule. Continuing education programs must be developed that prevent deterioration of necessary skills.

The ECC segment of a communitywide emergency system is best provided through a stratified system of coronary care having three levels. At level 1 are the ECC units, which include basic and advanced *fixed* ECC units and basic and advanced *mobile* units capable of defibrillation.[22,23] At level 2 are the emergency care units, coronary care units, and intermediate care units capable of thrombolytic therapy[24,25] and intensive care. At level 3 are the tertiary care centers capable of coronary revascularization and other necessary interventions.

The Chain of Survival

In recent years many clinicians, administrators, and researchers have recognized the need to improve the total ECC system to optimize patient survival. Communities must identify weaknesses in the ECC system, implement modifications to strengthen the system, and optimize treatment for these critical patients.[26]

The central issue is whether a community's ECC system results in optimal patient survival. Achieving the optimal survival rate for out-of-hospital cardiac arrest in every community is the challenge now and in the future. However, what is optimal in one community may not be possible in all communities. Early reports of high survival rates in midsized cities provided the EMS prototype adopted by most communities.[27,28] The obstacles to providing care in rural and large metropolitan areas create different challenges for EMS systems.[29] Therefore, each community must examine and devise its own mechanisms to achieve the goal of optimal patient survival rates.

Survival of cardiac arrest depends on a series of critical interventions. If any of these critical actions is neglected or delayed, survival is unlikely. The American Heart Association (AHA) has adopted and supported the ECC systems concept for years.[30,31] The phrase "chain of survival"[32] provides a useful

metaphor for the elements of the ECC systems concept (Fig 3). The ECC systems concept summarizes the present understanding of the best approach to the treatment of persons with sudden cardiac death. The four links in this chain are early access to the EMS system, early CPR, early defibrillation, and early advanced cardiac care. Epidemiological and clinical research have established that effective ECC, whether prehospital or in hospital, depends on these strong links that are closely interdependent.[22,33-35]

The chain of survival concept underscores several important principles:

- If any one link in the chain is inadequate, survival rates will be poor. Weakness in system components is the major explanation for variability in survival rates reported during the past 20 years.[27]
- All links must be strong to ensure rapid defibrillation. Unfortunately, long call-to-defibrillation intervals are common. Shorter intervals are necessary to improve survival rates.[22,26]
- Since the chain of survival has many links, the effectiveness of a system cannot be tested by examining an individual link. Rather, the whole system must be tested. The survival-to-discharge rate has emerged as the "gold standard" for assessing the effectiveness of the treatment of cardiac arrest. Recently considerable progress has been made toward providing clear methodological guidelines for study design, uniform terminology, and reporting of results.[27,36,37] This progress should facilitate future research on CPR and implementation of the chain of survival in each community.

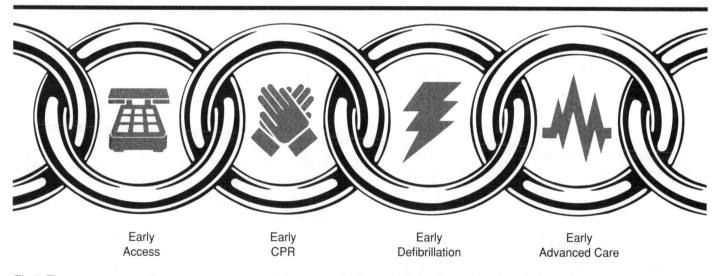

| Early | Early | Early | Early |
| Access | CPR | Defibrillation | Advanced Care |

Fig 3. The emergency cardiac care systems concept is displayed schematically by the "chain of survival" metaphor.

The First Link: Early Access

Early access encompasses the events initiated after the patient's collapse until the arrival of EMS personnel prepared to provide care. Recognition of early warning signs, such as chest pain and shortness of breath, that encourage patients to call 911 before collapse are key components of this link. With a cardiac arrest the major events that must occur rapidly include

- Early identification of patient collapse by a person who can activate the EMS system
- Recognition of unresponsiveness
- Rapid notification (usually by telephone) of the EMS dispatchers before CPR is begun for an adult and after 1 minute of rescue support for the child and infant
- Rapid recognition by the dispatchers of a potential cardiac arrest
- Rapid dispatch instructions to available EMS responders (first-, second-, and third-tier EMS personnel) to guide them to the patient
- Rapid arrival of EMS responders at the address
- EMS responder arrival at the patient's side with all necessary equipment
- Identification of the arrested state

All of these must take place before defibrillation or advanced care can occur. Each event is therefore a vital part of the early access link. In most communities, responsibility for these events rests with the 911 telephone system, the EMS dispatch system, and the EMS responder system.

The 911 Telephone System. In the United States, widespread use of 911 has simplified and expedited emergency assistance. Nevertheless, there are many US communities without 911 service. A more recent development is the implementation of "enhanced 911" in many communities. This option automatically provides dispatchers with the caller's address and telephone number. Obtaining 911 service — preferably enhanced 911 — should be a top priority for all communities.

The EMS Dispatch System. Rapid emergency medical dispatch has emerged as a vital part of the early access link.[38-42] While the organization, structure, and protocols of EMS dispatchers may vary, most functions are similar.

A new responsibility for EMS dispatchers is providing dispatcher-directed CPR. Dispatchers offer instructions to the caller on how to perform CPR until the EMS responders arrive. This method has been shown in controlled trials to be feasible and effective.[43,44] All EMS dispatch systems must be able to immediately answer all emergency medical calls, rapidly determine the nature of the call, identify the closest and most appropriate EMS responder unit(s), dispatch the unit to the scene on average in less than 1 minute, provide critical information to EMS responders about the type of emergency, and offer telephone-assisted CPR instructions.

The EMS Responder System. The EMS responder system is usually composed of responders trained in both BLS and ACLS.[39] The system may be structured for either a one-tier or a multi-tier level of response.[45] Most one-tier systems use ACLS-trained (paramedic) responders, although some one-tier systems provide only BLS. Two-tier systems generally provide first-responder units staffed with emergency medical technicians (EMTs) or firefighters close to the scene,[39] followed by the second tier of ACLS responders. Two-tier systems in which the first responders are trained in early defibrillation are most effective in providing rapid ACLS.[28,46]

Once dispatched, EMS responders must quickly reach the site of the cardiac arrest, locate the patient, and arrive at the patient's side with all necessary equipment.

The Second Link: Early CPR

CPR is most effective when started immediately after the victim's collapse. In almost all clinical studies, bystander CPR has been shown to have significant positive effect on survival.[10,29,47-49] The one possible exception to this is a situation in which the call-to-defibrillation interval is extremely short.[50] Bystander CPR is the best treatment that a cardiac arrest patient can receive until the arrival of a defibrillator and ACLS care.[10, 47-49] Training in basic CPR also teaches citizens how to gain access to the EMS system more efficiently, thus shortening the time to defibrillation. Bystander CPR rarely causes significant injury to victims, even when started inappropriately on people not in cardiac arrest.[22]

Communitywide CPR programs should be developed wherever possible, including schools, military bases, housing complexes, workplaces, and public buildings. Communities need to remove any barriers that discourage citizens from learning and performing CPR.

Although bystander CPR is clearly of value, it is only temporizing and loses its value if the next links (early defibrillation and early ACLS) do not rapidly follow. Therefore, for an adult victim, the bystander should determine unresponsiveness, call 911 for help, and then initiate CPR. Communities must target groups most likely to observe cardiac arrest or have the opportunity to perform bystander CPR. They should also place a priority on activation of the EMS system. The dispatcher should be told "CPR is in progress." A single, unassisted rescuer with an adult victim should activate the EMS system after establishing unresponsiveness. In a pediatric arrest, the EMS system should be activated after the trained rescuer provides 1 minute of rescue support.

The Third Link: Early Defibrillation

Early defibrillation is the link in the chain of survival most likely to improve survival rates.[22,51-57] The placement of automated external defibrillators (AEDs) in the hands of large numbers of people trained in their use may be the key intervention for increasing the survival chances for out-of-hospital cardiac arrest patients (Table 1).[57] The AHA strongly endorses the position that every emergency vehicle that may transport cardiac arrest patients be equipped with a defibrillator and that emergency personnel be trained to use and permitted to operate this device.[23] To assist in achieving this goal, the International Association of Fire Chiefs has endorsed equipping every fire suppression unit in the United States with an AED.[58]

Several options exist for rapid defibrillation. Defibrillation can be performed with manual, automatic, or semiautomatic external defibrillators. Manual defibrillation requires interpretation of a monitor or rhythm strip and is usually performed by responders trained in ACLS. Even so, manual defibrillation by EMTs trained to recognize ventricular fibrillation improves survival.[51,52] Defibrillation using automatic, automatic advisory, or semiautomatic external defibrillators is also effective.[56] These devices analyze the rhythm and either automatically defibrillate or advise the operator to defibrillate. The widespread effectiveness and demonstrated safety of the AED have made it acceptable for nonmedical professionals to effectively operate the device for use with adult victims. Such persons must still be trained in CPR and the use of defibrillators. In the near future, more creative use of AEDs by nonprofessionals may result in improved survival rates.[22]

When EMS resources are limited, defibrillators should be prioritized over many other medical devices, such as automatic transport ventilators or mobile 12-lead electrocardiogram (ECG) units.

Participants in the 1992 National Conference on CPR and ECC recommended that

- AEDs be widely available to appropriately trained people
- All fire-fighting units that perform CPR and first aid be equipped with and trained to operate AEDs
- AEDs be placed in gathering places of more than 10 000 people
- Legislation be enacted to allow all EMS personnel to perform early defibrillation

The Fourth Link: Early ACLS

Early ACLS provided by paramedics at the scene is another critical link in the management of cardiac arrest. ACLS brings equipment to support ventilation, establishes intravenous access, administers drugs, controls arrhythmias, and stabilizes the victim for transport.

EMS System Evaluation

EMS systems should have sufficient staffing to provide a minimum of two rescuers trained in ACLS to respond to the emergency. However, because of the difficulties in treating cardiac arrest in the field, additional responders should be present. In systems that have attained survival rates higher than 20% for patients with ventricular fibrillation, the response teams have a minimum of two ACLS providers plus a minimum of two BLS personnel at the scene.[59] Most experts agree that four responders (at least two trained in ACLS and two trained in BLS) are the minimum required to provide ACLS to cardiac arrest victims. Although not every EMS system can attain this level of response, every system should actively pursue this goal.

The best way to evaluate the strength of the chain of survival is to assess the survival rates achieved by the system. The cost of data collection for a system may be significant. However, it is only through evaluation that systems can routinely improve their services. All ECC systems should assess their performance

Table 1. Effectiveness of Early Defibrillation Programs[51]

Location	Before early defibrillation	After early defibrillation	Odds ratio for improved survival
King County, Washington	7	26 (10/38)	3.7
Iowa	3 (1/31)	19 (12/64)	6.3
SE Minnesota	4 (1/27)	17 (6/36)	4.3
NE Minnesota	2 (3/118)	10 (8/81)	5.0
Wisconsin	4 (32/893)	11 (33/304)	2.8

Values are percent surviving and, in parentheses, how many patients had ventricular fibrillation.

through an ongoing evaluation process. For evaluation data to be meaningful, it is necessary to compare EMS systems. This, in turn, requires standardized definitions and terms of reference (Table 2). Until recently, uniform terminology has not been available, producing a cardiac arrest Tower of Babel.[27] Reported survival rates in the literature range from 2% to 44%. It is not yet understood whether these profound variations are due to differences in population, treatment protocol, system organization, rescuer skills, or reporting practices.

There is now international consensus on the importance of using standard terminology and methods to evaluate survival and the chain of survival.[37] Clear, unambiguous terminology has been created, a uniform method of reporting data has been established, and methods for cardiac arrest research have been improved.[27,36,37] Improving the ECC system, however, first requires an accurate measurement of the survival rate for each community. This can be achieved by implementing the following recommendations:

Table 2. Definitions and Terminology in Emergency Cardiac Care (ECC)[37]

Cardiac arrest. — Cardiac arrest is the cessation of cardiac mechanical activity. It is a clinical diagnosis, confirmed by unresponsiveness, absence of detectable pulse, and apnea (or agonal respirations).

Cardiopulmonary resuscitation (CPR). — In its broadest sense CPR refers to attempting any of the maneuvers and techniques used to restore spontaneous circulation.

Basic CPR. — Basic CPR is the attempt to restore spontaneous circulation using the techniques of chest wall compressions and pulmonary ventilation.

Bystander CPR, layperson CPR, or citizen CPR. — These terms are synonymous; however, bystander CPR is preferred. Bystander CPR is an attempt at basic CPR provided by a person not at that moment part of the organized emergency response system.

Basic life support (BLS). — BLS is the phase of ECC that includes recognition of cardiac arrest, access to the EMS system, and basic CPR. It may also refer to the educational program in these subjects.

Advanced CPR or advanced cardiac life support (ACLS). — These terms refer to attempts at restoration of spontaneous circulation using basic CPR plus advanced airway management, endotracheal intubation, defibrillation, and intravenous medications. ACLS may also refer to the educational program that provides guidelines for these techniques.

Emergency medical services (EMS) or emergency personnel. — Persons who respond to medical emergencies in an official capacity are emergency (or EMS) personnel. The EMS system has two major functional divisions: EMS dispatchers and EMS responders.

EMS dispatchers. — EMS personnel responsible for dispatching EMS responders to the scene of medical emergencies and providing telephone instructions to bystanders at the scene while professionals are en route.

EMS responders. — EMS personnel who respond to medical emergencies by going to the scene in an emergency vehicle. They may be first responders, second responders, or third responders, depending on the EMS system. They may be trained in ACLS or BLS. All should be capable of performing defibrillation. Emergency medical technician (EMT) usually denotes BLS training. Paramedic or EMT-P usually denotes ACLS training.

ECC system. — The ECC system refers to all aspects of ECC, including that rendered by emergency personnel. The extended ECC system also includes bystander CPR, rapid activation of the EMS system, emergency departments, intensive care units, cardiac rehabilitation, cardiac prevention programs, BLS and ACLS training programs, and citizen defibrillation.

Chain of survival. — The chain of survival is a metaphor to communicate the interdependence of a community's emergency response to cardiac arrest. This response is composed of four links: early access, early CPR, early defibrillation, and early ACLS. With a weak or missing link the result will be poor chances of survival, despite excellence in the rest of the ECC system.

Presumed cardiac cause. — Cardiac arrest due to presumed cardiac cause is the major focus of ECC. When reporting cardiac outcome data, studies of cardiac arrest should exclude arrests due to obvious noncardiac causes. Because of practical considerations (lack of autopsy information, cost), all arrests are considered to be of cardiac cause unless an obvious noncardiac cause can be identified. Common noncardiac diagnoses that should be separated during analysis of cardiac arrest outcome include sudden infant death syndrome, drug overdose, suicide, drowning, trauma, exsanguination, and terminal states of illness.

Time intervals. — The Utstein recommendations have provided a rational nomenclature for important time intervals. Time intervals should be reported as the A-to-B interval, which represents the period that begins at time point A and ends at time point B. These are more informative than imprecise terms like "downtime" or "response time." The following terms, for example, are suggested:

911-call-to-dispatch interval. — The interval from the time the call for help is first received by the 911 center until the time the emergency vehicle leaves for the scene.

Vehicle-dispatch-to-scene interval. — The interval from when the emergency vehicle departs for the scene until EMS responders indicate the vehicle has stopped at the scene or address. This does not include the time interval until emergency personnel arrive at the patient's side or the interval until defibrillation occurs.

Vehicle-at-scene-to-patient-access interval. — The interval from when the emergency response vehicle stops moving at the scene or address until EMS responders are at the side of the patient.

Call-to-defibrillation interval. — The interval from receipt of the call at the 911 center until the patient receives the first shock.

1. Develop an evaluation process in every ECC system.
2. Include an accurate assessment of survival rate using standardized nomenclature and reporting methods. This focus on quality improvement should identify practical goals given the structure and demographic characteristics of the local system; identify current performance, including the survival rate; identify gaps between goals and current performance; identify strategies to improve system performance; and evaluate whether performance improves with these modifications.
3. Design the evaluation specifically to benefit the local community. As a secondary interest, information should be shared regionally and nationally to help other communities develop optimal systems.
4. In assessments of survival, integrate into EMS systems evolving concepts of consensus terminology, data collection, system description, and CPR research methods.

Role of the American Heart Association

The AHA is the world's largest volunteer health organization. Its mission is the reduction of disability and death from cardiovascular diseases and stroke.

In 1963 the AHA established a Committee on Cardiopulmonary Resuscitation. It was expanded in 1971 to include ECC and became the Subcommittee on Emergency Cardiac Care. Pediatric resuscitation was added as a working group in 1978. In 1989 the ECC subcommittee gained committee status, and the working groups were elevated to subcommittees.

The goal of AHA CPR-ECC programs is to increase the number of persons knowledgeable about prevention of heart disease and preventable injuries and to educate the lay public and healthcare professionals about the emergency treatment of cardiac arrest and sudden cardiac death. The AHA provides support for control of cardiovascular disease through research, education, and community service programs. Its ECC training network is a structure for education that is effective and allows individuals in the community to participate in a variety of ways.

Many opportunities exist for volunteers to serve the AHA in development, communications, and program areas, including ECC. Contact your AHA affiliate if you are interested in helping the AHA achieve its mission.

References

1. *Morbidity and Mortality Chartbook on Cardiovascular, Lung and Blood Diseases 1990.* Bethesda, Md: National Heart, Lung, and Blood Institute; 1990.
2. *Heart and Stroke Facts: 1994 Statistical Supplement.* Dallas, Tex: American Heart Association; 1993.
3. Goldman L, Cook EF. The decline in ischemic heart disease mortality rates: an analysis of the comparative effects of medical interventions and changes in lifestyle. *Ann Intern Med.* 1984;101:825-836.
4. Bainton CR, Peterson DR. Deaths from coronary heart disease in persons 50 years of age and younger: a community-wide study. *N Engl J Med.* 1963;268:569-575.
5. Kuller L, Lilienfeld A, Fisher R. Sudden and unexpected deaths in young adults: an epidemiological study. *JAMA.* 1966;198:248-252.
6. Kuller L, Lilienfeld A, Fisher R. Epidemiological study of sudden and unexpected deaths due to arteriosclerotic heart disease. *Circulation.* 1966;34:1056-1068.
7. McNeilly RH, Pemberton J. Duration of last attack in 998 fatal cases of coronary artery disease and its relation to possible cardiac resuscitation. *BMJ.* 1968;3:139-142.
8. Gordon T, Kannel WB. Premature mortality from coronary heart disease: the Framingham Study. *JAMA.* 1971;215:1617-1625.
9. Carveth SW. Eight-year experience with a stadium-based mobile coronary care unit. *Heart Lung.* 1974;3:770-774.
10. Cummins RO, Eisenberg MS. Prehospital cardiopulmonary resuscitation: is it effective? *JAMA.* 1985;253:2408-2412.
11. Shu CY. Mobile CCUs. *Hospitals.* 1971;45:14.
12. Kuller L, Cooper M, Perper J. Epidemiology of sudden death. *Arch Intern Med.* 1972;129:714-719.
13. Pantridge JF, Geddes JS. Cardiac arrest after myocardial infarction. *Lancet.* 1966;1:807-808.
14. Pantridge JF. The effect of early therapy on the hospital mortality from acute myocardial infarction. *Q J Med.* 1970;39:621-622.
15. Grace WJ, Chadbourn JA. The first hour in acute myocardial infarction. *Heart Lung.* 1974;3:736-741.
16. Division of Injury Control, Center for Environmental Health and Injury Control, Centers for Disease Control. Childhood injuries in the United States. *Am J Dis Child.* 1990;144:627-646.
17. Guyer B, Ellers B. Childhood injuries in the United States: mortality, morbidity, and cost. *Am J Dis Child.* 1990;144:649-652.
18. Rice DP, Mackenzie EJ, and Associates. *Cost of Injury in the United States: A Report to Congress.* San Francisco, Calif: Institute for Health and Aging, University of California and Injury Prevention Center, The Johns Hopkins University; 1989.
19. McIntyre KM. Cardiopulmonary resuscitation and the ultimate coronary care unit. *JAMA.* 1980;244:510-511.
20. Eisenberg MS, Bergner L, Hallstrom A. Cardiac resuscitation in the community: importance of rapid provision and implications for program planning. *JAMA.* 1979;241:1905-1907.
21. Thompson RG, Hallstrom AP, Cobb LA. Bystander-initiated cardiopulmonary resuscitation in the management of ventricular fibrillation. *Ann Intern Med.* 1979;90:737-740.
22. Cummins RO, Ornato JP, Thies WH, Pepe PE. Improving survival from sudden cardiac arrest: the 'chain of survival' concept. A statement for health professionals from the Advanced Cardiac Life Support Subcommittee and the Emergency Cardiac Care Committee, American Heart Association. *Circulation.* 1991;83:1833-1847.

23. Kerber RE. Statement on early defibrillation from the Emergency Cardiac Care Committee, American Heart Association. *Circulation.* 1991;83:2233.

24. ACC/AHA guidelines for the early management of patients with acute myocardial infarction. A report of the American College of Cardiology/American Heart Association Task Force on Assessment of Diagnostic and Therapeutic Cardiovascular Procedures. Special report. *Circulation.* 1990;82:664-707.

25. ACC/AHA guidelines for the early management of patients with acute myocardial infarction. A report of the American College of Cardiology/American Heart Association Task Force. Special report. *J Am Coll Cardiol.* 1990;16:249-292.

26. Weaver WD, Cobb LA, Hallstrom AP, Copass MK, Ray R, Emery M, Fahrenbruch C. Considerations for improving survival from out-of-hospital cardiac arrest. *Ann Emerg Med.* 1986;15:1181-1186.

27. Eisenberg MS, Cummins RO, Damon S, Larsen MP, Hearne TR. Survival rates from out-of-hospital cardiac arrest: recommendations for uniform definitions and data to report. *Ann Emerg Med.* 1990;19:1249-1259.

28. Eisenberg MS, Horwood BT, Cummins RO, Reynolds-Haertle R, Hearne TR. Cardiac arrest and resuscitation: a tale of 29 cities. *Ann Emerg Med.* 1990;19:179-186.

29. Becker LB, Ostrander MP, Barrett J, Kondos GT, CPR Chicago. Outcome of CPR in a large metropolitan area: where are the survivors? *Ann Emerg Med.* 1991;20:355-361.

30. Atkins JM. Emergency medical service systems in acute cardiac care: state of the art. *Circulation.* 1986;74(suppl IV): IV-4-IV-8.

31. American Heart Association. Standards and guidelines for cardiopulmonary resuscitation (CPR) and emergency cardiac care (ECC). *JAMA.* 1980;244:453-508.

32. Newman MM. The Chain of Survival concept takes hold. *J Emerg Med Serv.* 1989;14:11-13.

33. Eisenberg MS, Bergner L, Hallstrom AP. Paramedic programs and out-of-hospital cardiac arrest: I. Factors associated with successful resuscitation. *Am J Public Health.* 1979;69:31-38.

34. Eisenberg MS, Bergner L, Hallstrom AP. Paramedic programs and out-of-hospital cardiac arrest: II. Impact on community mortality. *Am J Public Health.* 1979;69:39-42.

35. Eisenberg MS, Copass MK, Hallstrom AP, Cobb LA, Bergner L. Management of out-of-hospital cardiac arrest: failure of basic emergency medical technician services. *JAMA.* 1980;2243:1049-1051.

36. Jastremski MS. In-hospital cardiac arrest. *Ann Emerg Med.* 1993;22:113-117.

37. Cummins RO, Chamberlain DA, Abramson NS, Allen M, Baskett PJ, Becker L, Bossaert L, Delooz HH, Dick WF, Eisenberg MS, Evans TR, Holmberg S, Kerber R, Mullie A, Ornato JP, Sandoe E, Skulberg A, Tunstall-Pedoe H, Swanson R, Thies WH. Recommended guidelines for uniform reporting of data from out-of-hospital cardiac arrest: the Utstein Style. A statement for health professionals from a task force of the American Heart Council, the Heart and Stroke Foundation of Canada, and the Australian Resuscitation Council. *Circulation.* 1991;84:960-975.

38. Clawson JJ. Emergency medical dispatching. In: Roush WR, ed. *Principles of EMS Systems: A Comprehensive Text for Physicians.* Dallas, Tex: American College of Emergency Physicians; 1989:119-133.

39. Pepe PE, Almaguer DR. Emergency medical services personnel and ground transport vehicles. *Probl Crit Care.* 1990;4: 470-476.

40. Curka PA, Pepe PE, Ginger VF, Sherrard RC. Computer-aided EMS priority dispatch: ability of a computed triage system to safely spare paramedics from responses not requiring advanced life support. *Ann Emerg Med.* 1991;20:446. Abstract.

41. Clawson JJ. Emergency medical dispatch. In: Kuehl A, ed. *EMS Medical Directors' Handbook.* St Louis, Mo: Mosby Year Book; 1989:59-90.

42. National Association of EMS Physicians. Emergency medical dispatching: a position paper. *Prehosp Disaster Med.* 1989;4: 163-166.

43. Eisenberg MS, Hallstrom AP, Carter WB, Cummins RO, Bergner L, Pierce J. Emergency CPR instruction via telephone. *Am J Public Health.* 1985;75:47-50.

44. Kellermann AL, Hackman BB, Somes G. Dispatcher-assisted cardiopulmonary resuscitation: validation of efficacy. *Circulation.* 1989;80:1231-1239.

45. Braun O, McCallion R, Fazackerley J. Characteristics of midsized urban EMS systems. *Ann Emerg Med.* 1990;19: 536-546.

46. Pepe PE, Bonnin MJ, Almaguer DR, et al. The effect of tiered system implementation on sudden death survival rates. *Prehosp Disaster Med.* 1989;4:71. Abstract.

47. Ritter G, Wolfe RA, Goldstein S, Landis JR, Vasu CM, Acheson A, Leighton R, Medendrop SV. The effect of bystander CPR on survival of out-of-hospital cardiac arrest victims. *Am Heart J.* 1985;110:932-937.

48. Bossaert L, Van Hoeyweghen R. Bystander cardiopulmonary resuscitation (CPR) in out-of-hospital cardiac arrest: the Cerebral Resuscitation Study Group. *Resuscitation.* 1989;17(suppl):S55-S69.

49. Cummins RO, Eisenberg MS, Hallstrom AP, Litwin PE. Survival of out-of-hospital cardiac arrest with early initiation of cardiopulmonary resuscitation. *Am J Emerg Med.* 1985;3: 114-119.

50. Troiano P, Masaryk J, Stueven HA, Olson D, Barthell E, Waite EM. The effect of bystander CPR on neurologic outcome in survivors of prehospital cardiac arrests. *Resuscitation.* 1989;17:91-98.

51. Cummins RO. From concept to standard-of-care? Review of the clinical experience with automated external defibrillators. *Ann Emerg Med.* 1989;18:1269-1275.

52. Stults KR, Brown DD, Kerber RE. Efficacy of an automated external defibrillator in the management of out-of-hospital cardiac arrest: validation of the diagnostic algorithm and initial clinical experience in a rural environment. *Circulation.* 1986;73:701-709.

53. Weaver WD, Hill D, Fahrenbruch CE, Copass MK, Martin JS, Cobb LA, Hallstrom AP. Use of the automatic external defibrillator in the management of out-of-hospital cardiac arrest. *N Engl J Med.* 1988;319:661-666.

54. Wright D, James C, Marsden AK, Mackintosh AF. Defibrillation by ambulance staff who have had extended training. *BMJ.* 1989;299:96-97.

55. Paris PM. EMT-defibrillation: a recipe for saving lives. *Am J Emerg Med.* 1988;6:282-287.

56. Cummins RO, Thies W. Encouraging early defibrillation: the American Heart Association and automated external defibrillators. *Ann Emerg Med.* 1990;19:1245-1248.

57. Cobb LA, Eliastam M, Kerber RE, Melker R, Moses AJ, Newell L, Paraskos JA, Weaver WD, Weil M, Weisfeldt ML. Report of the American Heart Association Task Force on the Future of Cardiopulmonary Resuscitation. *Circulation.* 1992;85:2346-2355.

58. Murphy DM. Rapid defibrillation: fire service to lead the way. *J Emerg Med Serv.* 1987;12:67-71.

59. Pepe P. Advanced cardiac life support: state of the art. In: Vincent JL, ed. *Emergency and Intensive Care.* New York, NY: Springer-Verlag NY Inc; 1990:565-585.

Cardiopulmonary Functions and Actions for Survival

This chapter describes the anatomy (structure) and physiology (function) of the cardiovascular and respiratory systems, clinical manifestations of coronary heart diseases, and actions for survival.

The Cardiovascular and Respiratory Systems

Anatomy of the Cardiovascular System

The cardiovascular system comprises the heart, arteries, capillaries, and veins. The heart of an adult is not much larger than a fist. It lies in the center of the chest, behind the breastbone (sternum), in front of the backbone (thoracic spine), and above the diaphragm. Except for the area of the heart against the spine and a small strip down the center of the front of the heart, it is surrounded by lung (Fig 1).

The heart is a hollow organ. Its tough, muscular wall (myocardium) is surrounded by a sac (pericardium) and has a thin, strong lining (endocardium). A wall (septum) divides the heart cavity into "right" and "left" sides. Each side is divided again into an upper chamber (atrium) and a lower chamber (ventricle). Valves regulate the flow of blood through the heart chambers and (1) into the pulmonary artery and then to the lungs or (2) into the aorta and then to the rest of the body (Fig 2).

Physiology of the Heart

The function of the heart is to pump blood to the lungs and to the body. Arteries and veins carry the blood to and from the capillaries and the heart. At the capillary level oxygen and carbon dioxide are exchanged between the blood and the tissues. This process occurs in the lungs, the rest of the body, and the heart muscle itself.

All body cells require oxygen continuously to carry out normal functions. Carbon dioxide is produced as a waste product and must be eliminated from the body through the lungs.

The heart is really a double pump. One pump (the right side of the heart) receives blood that has just returned from the body after delivering oxygen to the body tissues. It pumps this dark, bluish-red blood to the lungs, where the blood rids itself of waste gas (carbon dioxide) and picks up a supply of oxygen, which turns it a bright red again. The second pump (the left side of the heart) forces blood through the great trunk artery (aorta) and into smaller arteries, which distribute it to all parts of the body.

The adult heart at rest pumps 60 to 100 times per

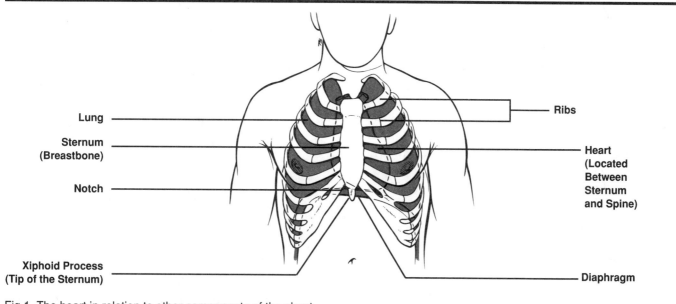

Fig 1. The heart in relation to other components of the chest.

Lung

Sternum (Breastbone)

Notch

Xiphoid Process (Tip of the Sternum)

Ribs

Heart (Located Between Sternum and Spine)

Diaphragm

The Heart and How It Works

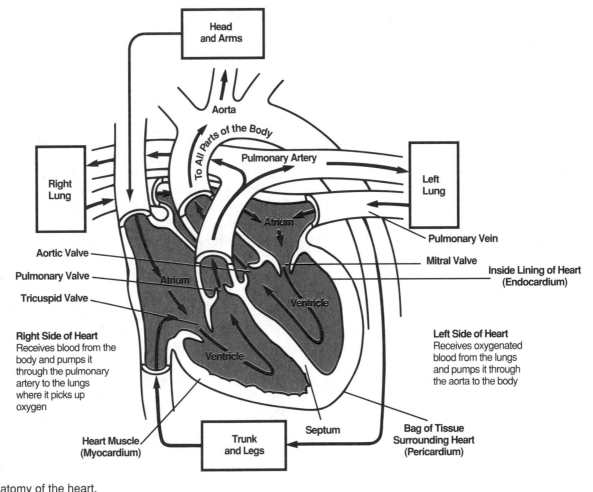

Fig 2. Anatomy of the heart.

minute. Each time the adult heart beats, it ejects about 2½ ounces of blood (approximately 70 milliliters). The heart pumps about 5 quarts (approximately 5 liters) of blood each minute during rest. During exercise the heart can pump up to 37 quarts (35 liters) each minute. The total blood volume of a 150-pound man is about 6 quarts (approximately 6 liters).

Each cardiac muscle contraction or heartbeat is initiated by an electrical impulse that arises from the natural pacemaker in the heart and is transmitted to the heart muscle by a specialized conduction system. The heart muscle contracts after it is stimulated by this electrical impulse. The contraction is followed by a period during which the electrical system and the heart muscle are recharged and made ready for the next beat. The heart has its own electrical pacemaker. Even if the heart is removed from the body, it will continue to beat if properly maintained. The heart rate, however, can be altered either by nerve impulses from the brain or by various substances in the blood that influence the pacemaker and the conduction system.

Anatomy of the Respiratory System

The respiratory system has four components (Fig 3):
- An *airway* from the outside of the body to the inside
- A *neuromuscular system*
- The lungs, comprising interconnecting air sacs, called *alveoli*
- The *arteries, capillaries,* and *veins*

1. The airway is composed of the following elements:
    - Upper airway
        — Nose and mouth
        — Pharynx (behind the tongue)
        — Larynx or voice box
    - Lower airway
        — Trachea or windpipe
        — Bronchi, one bronchus to the right lung and one to the left lung
        — Bronchioles, branches of the bronchi that terminate in the alveoli

The Respiratory System

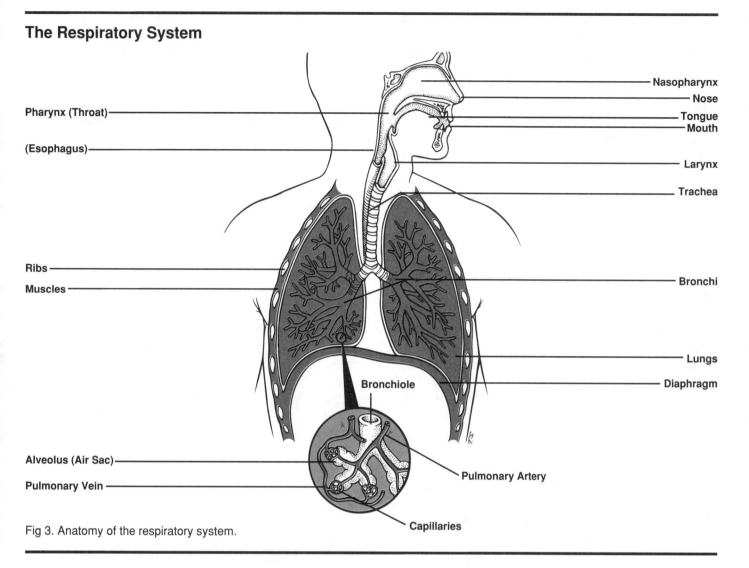

Fig 3. Anatomy of the respiratory system.

2. The neuromuscular system comprises the respiratory center in the brain, the nerves to the muscles of respiration, and the muscles of respiration. The chest cage, composed of the ribs supported in back by the spine and in front by the sternum, protects the lungs and allows breathing to occur. The major muscles of respiration are

   • The large sheetlike diaphragm attached to the margin of the lower ribs, which extends from front to back and separates the chest cavity from the abdominal cavity
   • The muscles between the ribs (the intercostal muscles)
   • Some of the muscles of the neck and shoulder girdle

3. The alveoli, millions of tiny air sacs that hold carbon dioxide and oxygen, are lined by a membrane. On the other side of the membrane is a fine network of capillaries. The alveoli, with their associated capillaries, are the basic lung units.

4. The pulmonary arteries carry blood, with low oxygen content, from the right heart. The capillaries surround the alveoli. The pulmonary veins carry blood, with high oxygen content, back to the left heart.

Physiology of the Respiratory System

The function of the respiratory system is to bring oxygen from the outside air into the blood and to eliminate carbon dioxide from the body. The cells of the body continuously need oxygen to function. As a result of using this oxygen, carbon dioxide is produced. Unless oxygen is continually supplied and carbon dioxide is continually eliminated from the body, death will result.

The cardiovascular system transports oxygen from the lungs to the cells of the body and transports carbon dioxide from the cells to the lungs for elimination.

In most healthy persons the levels of oxygen and

carbon dioxide in the blood remain relatively constant. The stimulus to breathe comes from the respiratory center in the brain, but the primary stimulus for altering the depth and rate of breaths is the level of carbon dioxide in the arterial blood. As this level rises, the respiratory center in the brain sends an increasing number of signals by way of nerves to the muscles of respiration. The breathing rate and depth are increased until the level of carbon dioxide falls, and then the breathing rate slows. There is a constant feedback loop between the carbon dioxide level and the rate and depth of respiration. Thus the blood level of carbon dioxide is maintained in a narrow range.

At the level of the alveoli, oxygen from the air passes into the blood through the alveolar and capillary walls, and carbon dioxide passes in the opposite direction.

Atmospheric air contains about 21% oxygen and negligible amounts of carbon dioxide. Because only about a quarter of the oxygen in the inhaled air is taken up by the blood in the lungs during respiration, exhaled air still contains significant oxygen (about 16%) as well as a small amount of added carbon dioxide (5%) and water vapor. In CPR, the exhaled air of rescue breaths contains enough oxygen to support the life of the victim.

Inspiration (breathing in) is an active process. As the intercostal muscles contract, they elevate the ribs; as the diaphragm contracts, it descends toward the abdominal cavity. The lungs expand and the pressure within the lungs becomes less than that outside of the chest. The difference in pressure draws air into the airways and lungs. Expiration is generally a passive process. As the muscles relax, the ribs descend and the diaphragm rises, thereby decreasing the capacity of the chest cavity. The elastic lung passively becomes smaller, and the air inside the lung moves out.

Respiratory Arrest and Insufficiency

Respiratory arrest refers to the absence of breathing. Respiratory insufficiency implies that although breathing may be present, it is inadequate to maintain normal levels of oxygen and carbon dioxide in the blood.

Airway Obstruction

The obstructed airway is discussed in detail in chapter 4. The most common cause of airway obstruction is occlusion by upper airway structures such as the tongue and epiglottis, a fingerlike structure near the back of the throat. Any condition that leads to unconsciousness or loss of tone in the muscles of the jaw can cause the tongue (or epiglottis) to fall toward the back of the throat and obstruct the airway.[1] See chapter 4, Fig 4.

Foreign-body obstruction of the airway accounted for 3805 deaths in 1988.[2] The need for proper emergency airway management in cases of foreign-body obstruction is of key importance for safety in homes, restaurants, and other public places. See chapter 4.

Central Respiratory Arrest

The respiratory center in the brain must function for respiration to occur. It is severely affected by inadequate blood flow to the brain, as occurs in stroke (a condition caused by interruption of the blood supply to an area of the brain), shock, or cardiac arrest. Within a few seconds after the heart ceases to beat, respiration will cease. In fact, any condition that leads to inadequate oxygenation of blood, despite adequate blood flow to the brain, can lead to respiratory arrest. This includes drug overdose, use of narcotics and barbiturates, head trauma, and diseases or injuries that interfere with normal contraction of the muscles of respiration.

Coronary Artery Disease

Definition of Terms

Arteriosclerosis, commonly called "hardening of the arteries," includes a variety of conditions that cause the artery walls to thicken and lose elasticity.

Atherosclerosis is a form of arteriosclerosis in which the inner layers of artery walls become thick and irregular because of deposits of a fatty substance. As the interior walls of arteries become lined with layers of these deposits, the arteries become narrowed and the flow of blood through the arteries is reduced.

Coronary artery disease (CAD) is the presence of atherosclerosis in the coronary arteries.

Coronary heart disease (CHD) is coronary artery disease plus the presence of symptoms as manifested by angina (specific chest pain) or a history of acute myocardial infarction. The term *atherosclerotic heart disease* is synonymous with coronary heart disease.

Ischemic heart disease is a more general term that includes all causes of myocardial ischemia (poor blood supply to the heart muscle).

Pathology and Natural History

Atherosclerosis is a slow, progressive disease that may have its beginnings early in life. Significant disease may be present before the age of 20. Long before the function of the heart muscle is impaired, there is an asymptomatic period when risk factor modification may halt or reverse the process. The inner portion of the arterial wall becomes thickened with deposits of fats (lipid, cholesterol) and eventually calcium. The result is a gradual narrowing of the arterial lumen (Fig 4). When the blood flow is severely reduced by atherosclerosis, a clot can form as blood trickles and sludges through the narrowed vessel, causing a sudden, complete stoppage of blood flow.[3] Injury to the heart muscle occurs because of this decrease or interruption of blood flow, creating an imbalance between the demand of the heart muscle for oxygen and the ability of the narrowed coronary artery to meet that demand.

Atherosclerosis is a generalized disease process that may involve arteries in different areas, such as the heart (leading to a heart attack), the brain (leading to a stroke), or the legs (leading to pain precipitated by walking or leg cramps during exercise).

Clinical Manifestations of Coronary Heart Disease

Persons with coronary artery disease may show no signs or signals of heart disease (asymptomatic) or have signs that do suggest coronary heart disease (symptomatic). In a person with asymptomatic CAD (Fig 5), coronary artery narrowing progresses over

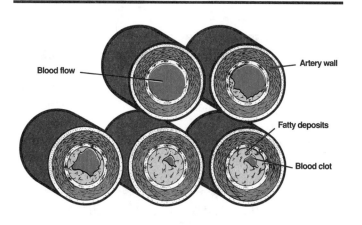

Fig 4. Progressive atherosclerotic buildup on artery walls with final stoppage of flow due to blood clot formation.

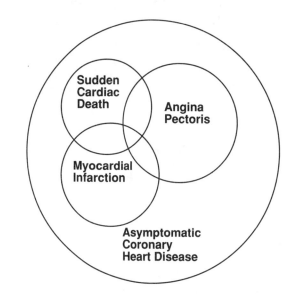

Fig 5. Clinical manifestations of coronary heart disease.

time. This is the period before enough decrease in blood supply occurs to produce symptoms of heart disease. Symptomatic CHD can manifest as chest discomfort (angina pectoris), a heart attack (myocardial infarction), or sudden death. Occasionally some people, especially those with diabetes, may have severe CHD on testing but otherwise have no symptoms. This is known as *silent ischemia*. Such patients are more likely to die or have a heart attack (as compared with those without silent ischemia).

Angina Pectoris

Angina pectoris, a common symptom of CHD, is a transient pain or discomfort due to a temporary lack of adequate blood supply to the heart muscle. The pain may be located in the center of the chest or it may be more diffuse, ie, throughout the front of the chest. It is usually described as being crushing, pressing, constricting, oppressive, or heavy (Fig 6). It may spread to one (more often the left) or both shoulders and/or arms or to the neck, jaw, back, or upper midportion of the abdomen (epigastrium). Discomfort occurring primarily in the arms, shoulders, neck, jaw, back, or epigastrium without anterior chest discomfort may also be a manifestation of angina. It is a steady discomfort, often brought on by any factor that increases the heart rate, including exercise, unusual exertion, and emotional or psychological stress. It commonly lasts from 2 to 15 minutes. The most frequent cause of angina is

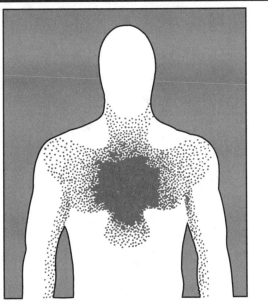

Fig 6. Intensity and location of pain as a symptom of coronary heart disease.

coronary atherosclerosis. As the severity of the coronary narrowing increases, the amount of exertion needed to bring on angina decreases. Angina is usually promptly relieved by rest or nitroglycerin. With severe CHD or a few days or weeks before a heart attack, angina may occur at rest or may even awaken someone from sleep.

Angina pectoris that is either new, worsening in severity (eg, more frequent, lasting longer, responding less to nitroglycerin or rest), or coming on at rest is called *unstable angina*. Patients with this form of angina are at high risk for acute myocardial infarction and should be hospitalized immediately.

Acute Myocardial Infarction (Heart Attack)

A heart attack occurs when an area of the heart muscle is deprived of blood (oxygen) for a prolonged period (usually more than 20 to 30 minutes). It usually results from severe narrowing or complete blockage of a diseased coronary artery and results in death of the heart muscle cells supplied by that artery. Blood vessel spasm (either spontaneous or secondary to drugs such as cocaine) can also result in a heart attack. The heart attack in turn may lead to altered electrical rhythms, including ventricular fibrillation. The usual symptom (signal) of a heart attack is a severe pressure or discomfort in the chest that persists for several minutes (more than 15 to 20 minutes) and is not relieved promptly by rest or nitroglycerin. In women and older persons, however, such typical symptoms occur less frequently.

Definition

Acute myocardial infarction means death of a part of the heart muscle due to inadequate oxygen and is another term for heart attack. Inadequate blood (oxygen) supply can be due to a clot in the coronary artery or narrowing due to atherosclerotic plaque. *Coronary* and *coronary thrombosis* are other terms for a heart attack.

Precipitating Events

In a study of patient activity at the onset of myocardial infarction, 59% were either at rest or asleep whereas 31% were involved in mild to moderate, or usual, exercise.[4] Emotional stress and life events with a powerful personal impact (eg, death of a significant other person, divorce, or loss of job) continue to be observed commonly before myocardial infarction and may be correlated.[5,6] Illicit drugs such as cocaine have clearly been shown to cause heart attacks and ventricular arrhythmias.

Warning Signs

- Chest discomfort is the most important signal of a heart attack. The discomfort is similar to angina in location, character, and radiation but is usually more intense, lasts considerably longer, and is not relieved by rest or nitroglycerin.
- Other signs may include sweating, nausea, or shortness of breath.
- A feeling of weakness may accompany chest discomfort.
- Be alert to the fact that
  — The discomfort may not be very severe, and the person may only have severe shortness of breath
  — The person does not necessarily have to "look bad" or have all the symptoms before action is taken
  — Stabbing, momentary twinges of pain are usually not signals of a heart attack
- The signals can occur in either sex, even in young adults, at any time and in any place.
- Do not be deceived by the patient's describing the discomfort as "sharp." This term is ambiguous. Some patients use the term to mean "stabbing" in quality whereas others use the term to mean "intense."

Actions for Survival

Many deaths from heart attack occur before victims reach the hospital. A great number of these fatalities could be prevented if the victim responded quickly, preferably within the first 2 minutes after the onset of the signs and signals. The usual cause of death in a heart attack is ventricular fibrillation.

Prevention is the best medicine, but despite efforts to educate the public about risk factors and early warning signals of heart attack, the rate of death from this major killer remains at an appalling level. More than half of all heart attack victims die outside the hospital, most within 2 hours of initial symptoms. It is essential to know and be able to recognize the signals of heart attack.

The initial treatment should be to have the patient rest quietly. Since both angina pectoris and heart attack are caused by a lack of adequate blood supply to the heart, activity must be kept at a minimum. When heart rate or blood pressure increases, such as during activity, the heart requires more oxygen. Rest keeps these at a minimum. The victim should be allowed to either lie down or sit up, whichever allows the most comfort and easiest breathing.

The victim's first tendency is to deny the possibility of a heart attack with such rationalizations as the following: *It's indigestion or something I ate. It can't happen to me. I'm too healthy. I don't want to bother my doctor. I'm under no strain. I don't want to frighten anyone. I'll take a home remedy. I'll feel ridiculous if it isn't a heart attack.* When the victim starts looking for reasons why he or she can't be having a heart attack, it is a signal for positive action.

If the typical chest discomfort lasts for more than a few minutes, emergency action should be initiated, unless the patient is a known heart patient whose physician has given instructions to take nitroglycerin first. Nitroglycerin tablets or spray under the tongue or as a patch or ointment on the skin may relieve the pain of angina pectoris. Since nitroglycerin lowers the blood pressure, it should be given with the victim sitting or lying down. It usually produces a stinging sensation under the tongue and may cause a headache.

Nitroglycerin tablets may be inactivated by age and light. It is best to keep a fresh supply in a dark place and carry only a few tablets in a small, dark bottle, changing to fresh tablets every month or so.

Even in known heart patients, if typical symptoms persist for 10 minutes despite rest and three nitroglycerin tablets, an emergency *action plan* should be followed (Fig 7).

For a person with unknown CHD:
1. Recognize the signals.
2. Stop activity and sit or lie down.
3. If pain persists for 5 minutes or more, phone first and call the EMS system. (Dial 911 or the local emergency number.) If the EMS system is not available, the patient should be taken immediately to the nearest hospital emergency department that provides 24-hour emergency care.

For a person with known CHD using nitroglycerin:
1. Recognize the signals.
2. Stop activity and sit or lie down.
3. Place one nitroglycerin tablet under the tongue or administer spray sublingually. Repeat at 3- to 5-minute intervals to a total dose of three tablets if discomfort is not relieved (ie, a maximum of 15 minutes). (Lay rescuers should be very cautious when administering a victim's nitroglycerin because the victim may already have taken some nitroglycerin and because tablet strengths may vary with the individual.)
4. If signals persist, phone first: call the EMS system. If an EMS system is not available, the victim should be taken immediately to the nearest hospital emergency department that provides 24-hour emergency care.

Everyone should have an emergency action plan at home and at work:
1. Know the appropriate emergency rescue service telephone number (usually 911).
2. Know the location of the nearest hospital emergency department that provides 24-hour emergency care.
3. Before the need for emergency services arises, discuss with the family physician the hospital of choice, distance to be traveled, and emergency facilities of hospitals under consideration.

Because the victim may deny the possibility of a heart attack, it is essential that the person nearest at the time activate emergency action and be prepared to render basic life support if necessary.

The person who is with someone having signals that last for 5 minutes or longer should act quickly. Expect a denial — but insist on taking prompt action:
1. Phone first! Call the EMS system. If EMS is not available:
2. Take the victim to the nearest hospital emergency department that provides 24-hour emergency care.
3. Be prepared to provide CPR (rescue breathing and chest compressions) if necessary. Training is the only way to be prepared.

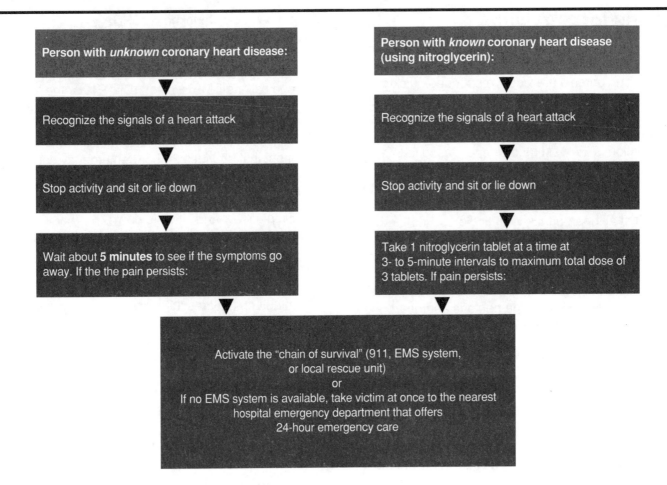

Fig 7. Emergency action plan for person with signals of heart attack.

Monitor the patient continuously by feeling the pulse. Electrocardiographic monitoring should be initiated as soon as possible. Oxygen should be administered, if available, by rescue personnel. Without warning, the patient may develop a rhythm disturbance that may cause cardiac arrest.

Sudden Cardiac Death (Cardiac Arrest)

Sudden death occurs when heartbeat and breathing stop abruptly or unexpectedly. Sudden cardiac death, or cardiac arrest, may occur as the initial and only manifestation of CHD. Sudden cardiac death may occur before any other symptom. It may also occur in persons with known CHD and especially during a heart attack. It most commonly occurs within 1 or 2 hours after the beginning of a heart attack.

The numerous noncardiac causes of sudden death are discussed in chapter 5.

Within seconds after cardiac arrest, the victim loses consciousness and breathing stops. During this early phase the victim may have a convulsion. The sooner circulation to the brain is restored, the greater the chance for full recovery of brain function. After 4 to 6 minutes of cardiac arrest, significant brain damage usually occurs. Children and victims of cold exposure or barbiturate overdose may recover normal brain function after longer periods of cardiac arrest.

Causes

Coronary heart disease is the most common cause of cardiac arrest. Yet any condition that interferes with the delivery of oxygen or blood to the heart or that causes irritation of the heart muscle itself may lead to cardiac arrest. These conditions include primary respiratory arrest, direct injury to the heart, drugs, or disturbances in heart rhythm. Since the heart does not require normal brain function to continue beating, brain injury by itself does not necessarily lead to cardiac arrest. It is generally the respiratory arrest resulting from brain injury that causes cardiac arrest. Once respiration ceases, however, the heart may continue to beat for several minutes until the oxygen level in the blood is so low that the heart stops beating.

In all victims of sudden death the direct cause of the cardiac arrest is ventricular fibrillation (a chaotic, uncoordinated quivering of the heart muscle), which results in the lack of an effective heartbeat.

Persons who have been successfully resuscitated from sudden death have often been found to have significant CHD, but many do not show evidence of a heart attack. In cardiac arrest due to ventricular fibrillation, the abnormal rhythm seldom can be converted to an effective heartbeat without electric defibrillation, although CPR may maintain vital organ perfusion for a few minutes. Defibrillation is the key to resuscitation and consists of the application of electric shock to the heart through the chest wall. The electric shock allows spontaneous coordinated electrical activity and effective heart function to return, thus producing an effective heartbeat. Defibrillation should be performed as soon as possible at the scene.

If CPR is initiated promptly and the patient is successfully and rapidly defibrillated, there is a good chance for survival. Early defibrillation is a vital link in the "chain of survival" and has been shown to significantly improve outcome in victims of out-of-hospital cardiac arrest.[7] It can be performed by minimally trained personnel using automated external defibrillators (AEDs). (See *Textbook of Advanced Cardiac Life Support,* chapter 4.) BLS providers working in healthcare systems that have AEDs are strongly encouraged to learn how to use them. AED courses can be freestanding and do not necessitate additional ACLS training.

References

1. Boidin MP. Airway patency in the unconscious patient. *Br J Anaesth.*1985;57:306-310.
2. *Vital Statistics of the United States, 1988.* Hyattsville, Md: National Center for Health Statistics;1988:2A.
3. DeWood MA, Spores J, Notske R, et al. Prevalence of total coronary occlusion during the early hours of transmural myocardial infarction. *N Engl J Med.* 1980;303:897-902.
4. Phipps C. Contributory causes of coronary thrombosis. *JAMA.* 1936;106:761-762.
5. Jenkins CD. Recent evidence supporting psychologic and social risk factors for coronary disease. *N Engl J Med.* 1976;294:1033-1038.
6. Rahe RH, Romo M, Bennett L, Siltanen P. Recent life changes, myocardial infarction, and abrupt coronary death: studies in Helsinki. *Arch Intern Med.* 1974;133:221-228.
7. Improving survival from sudden cardiac arrest: the 'chain of survival' concept. A statement for health professionals from the Advanced Cardiac Life Support Subcommittee and the Emergency Cardiac Care Committee, American Heart Association: Cummins RO, Ornato JP, Thies WH, Pepe PE. *Circulation.* 1991;83:1832-1847. Special report.

Risk Factors and Prudent Heart Living

Chapter 3

As investigators have searched for the causes of the "epidemic" of blood vessel diseases in the United States and many other countries, a consistent association has been found between specific conditions and behaviors and the development of blood vessel disease.[1,2] The "risk factor" concept developed from an awareness of these associations.

It is now well known that heart attack occurs much more frequently in persons who smoke and in those who have elevated blood cholesterol levels, elevated blood pressure, or a sedentary lifestyle. The greater the prevalence of such risk factors, the greater the likelihood of heart attack (or other blood vessel disease). The person who smokes one pack of cigarettes a day has a greater chance of heart attack and sudden death than a person who does not smoke, other things being equal.

Persons who have more than one risk factor may have many more times the chance of developing vascular disease than persons who have none.[3,4] For example, the person who has an abnormal serum cholesterol level and smokes two packs of cigarettes a day may have as much as 10 times the chance of having a heart attack as the person who has a normal blood cholesterol level and does not smoke. Fig 1 illustrates the incidence of the three major risk factors for coronary heart disease (CHD) — cigarette smoking, elevated blood cholesterol, and elevated blood pressure — and their relation to the likelihood of heart attack.

Risk Factors for Heart Attack

Risk Factors That Cannot Be Changed

Some risk factors cannot be modified or eliminated (Fig 2).

- **Heredity.** A history of premature CHD in siblings or parents suggests an increased susceptibility that may be a genetic factor.
- **Gender.** Women have a lower incidence of coronary atherosclerosis before menopause. The incidence increases significantly, however, in postmenopausal women, who also have a worse clinical course (as compared with men).
- **Age.** The death rate from CHD increases with age. However, nearly one in four deaths occurs in persons under age 65.

Risk Factors That Can Be Changed

Other risk factors are subject to modification or elimination (Fig 2).

Cigarette Smoke. The heart attack death rate among people who do not smoke is considerably lower than among people who do. For those who have given up the habit, the death rate eventually declines almost to that of people who have never smoked.[5-10]

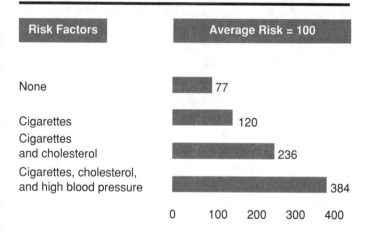

Risk Factors	Average Risk = 100
None	77
Cigarettes	120
Cigarettes and cholesterol	236
Cigarettes, cholesterol, and high blood pressure	384

Source: The Framingham, Mass, Heart Study

Fig 1. The danger of heart attack increases with the number of risk factors present.[1] For purposes of illustration, this chart uses an abnormal blood pressure level of 180 systolic and a cholesterol level of 310 in a 45-year-old man.

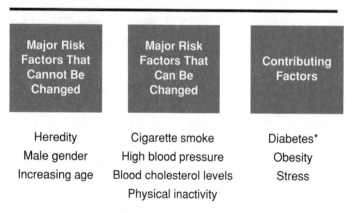

Major Risk Factors That Cannot Be Changed	Major Risk Factors That Can Be Changed	Contributing Factors
Heredity	Cigarette smoke	Diabetes*
Male gender	High blood pressure	Obesity
Increasing age	Blood cholesterol levels	Stress
	Physical inactivity	

Fig 2. Risk factors for heart disease. *The elevation in blood sugar level associated with diabetes can be controlled, but the increased risk of heart disease cannot be eliminated.

Passive smoking (inhalation of environmental tobacco smoke) has also been shown to be associated with an increased risk of smoking-related disease.[11,12] Hence all people — and especially those with other risk factors — should try to avoid exposure to passive smoke.

High Blood Pressure. A major risk factor for stroke and heart attack, high blood pressure usually has no specific symptoms but can be detected by a simple, painless test. A person with mild elevations of blood pressure often begins treatment with a program of weight reduction if overweight and salt (sodium) restriction before drugs are recommended.

High Blood Cholesterol Levels. Too much cholesterol can cause buildups on the walls of arteries, narrowing the passageway through which blood flows and leading to heart attack and stroke. A doctor can measure the amount of cholesterol in the blood with a simple test. Since the body gets cholesterol both through diet and by manufacturing it, a diet low in saturated fat and cholesterol will help lower the level of blood cholesterol if it is too high. Medications also are available that help maintain cholesterol levels within the normal range.

Physical Inactivity. Lack of exercise has been clearly established as a risk factor for heart attack. When combined with overeating, lack of exercise may lead to excess weight, which is an additional contributing factor. You should consult a doctor before you begin an exercise program or before you significantly increase your exercise level if you are over 40 years old.

Contributing Risk Factors

Other factors probably contribute indirectly to heart disease (Fig 2).

Diabetes. Diabetes appears most frequently during middle age and more often in people who are overweight. In its mild form, diabetes can go undetected for many years, but it can sharply increase a person's risk of heart attack, making control of other risk factors even more important. A doctor can detect diabetes and prescribe exercise and weight control programs, changes in eating habits, and drugs (if necessary) to keep it in check.

Obesity. In most cases obesity results simply from eating too much and exercising too little. Obesity places a heavy burden on the heart. It is associated with CHD primarily because of its role in increasing blood pressure and blood cholesterol and in precipitating diabetes. To help patients lose weight, doctors usually recommend a program that combines exercise with a low-calorie diet.

Excessive Stress. It is virtually impossible to define and measure a person's level of emotional and mental stress. All people feel stress, but they feel it in different amounts and react in different ways. Excessive stress over a long period may create health problems in some people. Most doctors agree that reduction of emotional stress will benefit the health of the average person.

Prudent Heart Living

Prudent heart living is a lifestyle that minimizes the risk of future heart disease. This lifestyle includes weight control, physical fitness, sensible dietary habits, avoidance of cigarette smoking, reduction of blood fats (such as cholesterol and triglycerides), and control of high blood pressure. This section on prudent heart living has been included for those interested in more detailed information about risk factors and their relation to heart disease.

The AHA also publishes a number of other materials concerning prudent heart living that may be useful as further information for the instructor and student. For more information contact your AHA affiliate.

A number of large studies have confirmed the effectiveness of risk factor modification in reducing cardiovascular morbidity and mortality.[13-24] Most authorities believe that risk factor reduction is an important part of a comprehensive approach to reducing cardiovascular illness and death in the community, especially among children and young adults.

While elevated cholesterol, cigarette smoking, and high blood pressure are considered the most significant risk factors, others have been identified. They include diabetes, obesity, male gender, heredity, advancing age, and a sedentary lifestyle. A strong family history of premature vascular disease and the presence of diabetes put people at higher risk for premature blood vessel disease. Persons at increased risk because of these factors should make special efforts to minimize their risk by eliminating smoking and by modifying high blood pressure.

Millions of Americans begin endangering their hearts at a comparatively early age by acquiring poor living habits. Children begin to overeat and develop a taste for foods high in salt and cholesterol and empty in calories. Some are not encouraged to get enough exercise, and watching television further limits play activity. The smoking habit frequently begins during early teen years, especially if parents smoke. By adulthood many Americans are overweight, lead sedentary lives, and smoke heavily. Many have high levels of cholesterol and triglycerides in their blood. High blood pressure is prevalent.

Most of the scientific evidence available today indicates that reducing risk factors may prevent many heart attacks. At the very least, reducing the risks can result in good general health and physical fitness and can benefit every member of the family. Children benefit most of all by learning the habits of prudent heart living early in life.

Eliminate Cigarette Smoking

In the United States cigarette smoking is a major cause of CHD in men.[25] It also markedly predisposes women who take oral contraceptives containing estrogens to cardiovascular disease. Because of the number of people in the population who smoke and the increased risk that smoking represents, "cigarette smoking should be considered the most important of the known modifiable risk factors for coronary heart disease in the United States."[25]

Overall, cigarette smokers experience a 70% greater CHD death rate than do nonsmokers. Heavy smokers (two or more packs per day) have CHD death rates between two and three times greater than those of nonsmokers. Cigarette smoking is a major independent risk factor, and it acts together with other risk factors (most notably elevated cholesterol and hypertension) to greatly increase the risk of CHD.

Before menopause women have lower rates for CHD than do men. Part of this difference is due to the fact that fewer women smoke, and those who do tend to smoke fewer cigarettes per day and inhale less deeply. However, among women who have smoking patterns comparable to those of men, CHD death rates are higher. Women who use oral contraceptives and who smoke increase their risk of myocardial infarction approximately 10-fold, compared with women who neither use oral contraceptives nor smoke.[26] In fact, recent data confirm that mortality rates after a heart attack are higher in women than in men.

Cigarette smoking has also been found to elevate the risk of sudden death significantly. Overall, smokers experience a two to four times greater risk of sudden death than nonsmokers. The risk appears to increase with the number of cigarettes smoked per day. It diminishes to almost normal with cessation of smoking.

Estimates are that in 1990 about 417 000 Americans died of smoking-related illnesses.[27] Nearly one fifth of deaths from cardiovascular disease are attributable to smoking.[27]

Unless smoking habits change, perhaps 10% of all persons now alive may die prematurely of heart disease attributable to their smoking behavior.[28] The total number of such premature deaths may exceed 24 million.

"Warning: The Surgeon General Has Determined That Cigarette Smoking Is Dangerous to Your Health." Many studies have shown that cigarette smokers have a greater risk of dying from a variety of diseases than do nonsmokers. If a smoker and a nonsmoker are victims of the same disease, the disease is more likely to be fatal to the smoker. The same studies indicate that people who give up smoking have a lower death rate from heart attack than do persistent smokers. After a period of years, the death rate of those who stop smoking is nearly as low as that of people who have never smoked. Some of the abnormal changes in lung tissue of heavy smokers have also been shown to gradually improve.

The earlier a person begins to smoke, the greater the risk to future health. There is considerable pressure on teenagers to smoke, and whether they resist may depend on the example set by their parents. In the majority of families where parents do not smoke, neither do the children.

Inhalation of environmental tobacco smoke, ie, "passive smoking," has also been associated with an increased risk of smoking-related disease. Public buildings, hospitals, and many restaurants and businesses have implemented firm nonsmoking policies. These efforts encourage patrons and employees to recognize risks for both active and passive smokers. Ongoing efforts in this public health area should lead to a decrease in the incidence of deaths and disability from cigarette smoking.

Control High Blood Pressure

As many as 50 million adults and children in the United States have high blood pressure.[27] It affects one in four American adults.[27]

Certain arteries in the body, called *arterioles,* regulate blood pressure. The manner in which arterioles control blood pressure is sometimes compared to the way a nozzle regulates water pressure in a hose. If the nozzle is turned to make the opening larger, less pressure is needed to force the water through the hose. If the nozzle is turned to make the opening narrower, or smaller, the pressure in the hose increases. Similarly, if the arterioles become narrower for any reason, the blood cannot easily pass through. This increases the blood pressure in the arteries and may overwork the heart. If the pressure increases above normal and stays there, the result is high blood pressure, or hypertension.

Primary, or essential, high blood pressure is the

most common type. Primary hypertension is of unknown origin, unlike secondary hypertension, which is caused by a disease, such as kidney disease.

Experts who have studied high blood pressure report that a tendency toward this disease is often found in families.[29] People whose parents had high blood pressure are more likely to develop it than people whose parents did not. If there is a family history of stroke or heart attack at an early age or if parents have high blood pressure, all members of the family should have regular blood pressure checks.

Primary high blood pressure cannot be cured, but it can usually be controlled. Uncontrolled high blood pressure adds to the workload of the heart and arteries. The heart, forced to work harder than normal over a long period, tends to enlarge. A slightly enlarged heart may function well, but a heart that is very much enlarged has a hard time keeping up with the demands made on it.

As people grow older, the arteries and their smaller branches, the arterioles, become hardened and less elastic. This process, arteriosclerosis, takes place gradually, even in people who do not have high blood pressure. However, high blood pressure tends to speed up the hardening.

The possibility of stroke is increased with high blood pressure and age. Uncontrolled high blood pressure can also affect the kidneys.

These effects on the heart, kidneys, and brain are called *end-organ damage.* This damage can be prevented or reduced if high blood pressure is treated early and continued.

Moderate elevations of blood pressure may be controlled by weight reduction and decreased sodium intake. The optimal degree of sodium reduction has not yet been completely established. Table salt is 40% sodium. Removing the salt shaker from the table and not adding salt while cooking can significantly reduce salt consumption. A physician's advice about weight reduction should be obtained. For persons with severe hypertension or mild to moderate hypertension not controlled by these measures, antihypertensive drugs can be used. Blood pressure needs to be controlled long term.

Decrease Blood Cholesterol Levels

Cholesterol is the main lipidlike (fat) component of the atherosclerotic deposits. An elevation of the total blood cholesterol level (hypercholesterolemia) has been consistently associated with CHD.[30] Although hypercholesterolemia is sometimes a family trait, it is most often due to environmental factors, the most

influential being diet. Studies in humans have shown that the serum cholesterol level can be raised in most people by ingestion of saturated fat and cholesterol and lowered by substantially reducing this intake.

The National Heart, Lung, and Blood Institute investigated the effect of cholesterol lowering on risk of CHD in men for 7 years in the Coronary Primary Prevention Trial.[31,32] Two groups were studied, both receiving a diet that lowered cholesterol by 4%. One group received the drug cholestyramine, which lowered cholesterol by an additional 8.5%. The group with the lower cholesterol level had a 24% reduction in CHD and a 19% reduction in heart attacks. This is the first conclusive evidence that a reduction in cholesterol by drug treatment can decrease the incidence of CHD and heart attack. An elevation of serum triglyceride (the main fatty substance in the fluid portion of blood) is also associated with an increased risk of CHD.

Cholesterol is a substance that is manufactured by the body but is also present in the animal products we eat. It is found in especially large amounts in egg yolk and organ meats. Shrimp and lobster are moderately high in cholesterol, though low in saturated fat, and hence they represent "better" eating choices. Excess cholesterol is deposited in the arteries and may lead to atherosclerosis.

Diets rich in saturated fats raise blood cholesterol levels in most people. The major sources of saturated fats are meat, animal fats, some vegetable oils (palm kernel oil, coconut oil, cocoa butter, and heavily hydrogenated margarines and shortenings), dairy products (whole milk, cream, butter, ice cream, and cheese), and bakery goods. Polyunsaturated fats and monounsaturated fats, on the other hand, tend to lower the level of cholesterol. The goal is to keep the total amount of fat, as well as saturated fat alone, low in the diet. By partially substituting polyunsaturated and monounsaturated fats for saturated fat and by increasing the amount of complex carbohydrates in the diet, it is possible to achieve the goal. The following points are illustrations of what these recommendations mean in terms of food:

- Eat fish or poultry for most meals, using no more than 6 ounces per day. When you do prepare red meat (beef, pork, lamb), use lean cuts, trim off excess fat, and serve small portions. Do not eat the skin of poultry.
- Cook with limited amounts of liquid vegetable oils and polyunsaturated, nonhydrogenated margarines (eg, canola, corn, cottonseed, soybean, and safflower products). Olive oil is a monounsaturated fat source.
- Use skim milk products.

- Eat no more than three egg yolks per week. Use egg substitutes in place of eggs.
- Use low-fat cooking methods, such as baking, broiling, and roasting. Avoid fried foods.

Changes in diet should never be drastic. Elimination of essential foods can be harmful. Fad diets that totally exclude one type of food from the diet can lead to additional health problems. However, with moderate changes in diet and careful monitoring of cholesterol and saturated fats, blood cholesterol can usually be kept at acceptable levels.

It is generally accepted that atherosclerosis may begin in childhood, progress through young adulthood, and become manifest only in middle age or later. It is therefore recommended that children more than 2 years old follow the same dietary guidelines recommended here for adults.[33]

Get More Exercise

Studies have shown that men who lead sedentary lives run a higher risk of heart attack than those who exercise regularly.[34-38] Studies have also suggested that a prudent exercise program is beneficial as part of a comprehensive risk reduction program.[39] Regular exercise can increase cardiovascular functional capacity and may decrease myocardial oxygen demand for any given level of physical activity. The risk of vigorous physical activity may be reduced by appropriate medical evaluation.

Exercise tones the muscles, stimulates the circulation, helps prevent obesity, and promotes a general feeling of well-being. Exercise can help control blood lipid abnormalities and diabetes. There is evidence to suggest that the survival rate of heart attack victims is higher in those who have exercised regularly than in those who have not.

People of all ages should develop a physically active lifestyle as part of a comprehensive program of heart disease prevention. Especially valuable are aerobic activities requiring movement of body weight over distance — walking, climbing stairs, running, cycling, swimming, and similar activities. Improvements in cardiovascular fitness appear to result from regular exercise of moderate intensity (50% to 75% of capacity) that is performed 15 to 30 minutes at least every other day. Vigorous exercise should be prescribed with caution for high-risk patients. Graded exercise tolerance tests, which may be used to help formulate a person's exercise prescription, should be performed under medical supervision.

Strenuous and unaccustomed activity occasionally brings on a heart attack in an apparently healthy person who has undiagnosed heart disease. Before someone over 40 years of age or with a known risk of cardiovascular disease undertakes an exercise program or engages in heavy physical labor, a physician should be consulted. An exercise test may be part of the evaluation of the person's physical condition. Physical activity should be increased gradually in any exercise program. If the physician indicates that the person is physically fit, introducing an enjoyable sport into the lifestyle can be beneficial.

Control Diabetes

Diabetes, or a familial tendency toward diabetes, is associated with an increased risk of CHD. The risk of CHD is twice as great in diabetic men and three times as great in diabetic women as in persons free of this disease. Diabetic women may have as great a mortality from CHD as nondiabetic men of the same age. The control of hyperglycemia (increased blood sugar) alone does not appear to reduce the risk that diabetes will adversely affect the large blood vessels.[40] The diabetic should pay close attention to the management of other commonly associated risk factors (hypercholesterolemia, hypertriglyceridemia, hypertension, and obesity).

Eliminate Obesity

Obesity is associated with an increased occurrence of CHD, particularly angina pectoris and sudden death, largely as a consequence of its influence on blood pressure, blood lipids, and the risk of diabetes.[41-44] There is evidence that obesity may directly contribute to CHD.[45-47] Few persons become obese without developing a less favorable coronary risk profile.

Most people reach their normal adult weight between the ages of 21 and 25. With each succeeding year, fewer calories are needed to maintain this weight. People in their 30s and 40s who eat as much as they did in their early 20s and who become physically less active will store the excess calories as body fat.

Life expectancy may be shorter for people who are markedly overweight. Middle-aged men who are significantly overweight have about three times the risk of a fatal heart attack as middle-aged men of normal weight. Obesity also means greater risk of hypertension and diabetes.

There is no quick, easy way to lose weight. Extreme reducing diets are best avoided because they usually exclude foods essential to good health. Even when these diets do lower weight, patterns of eating that will help maintain normal weight are not developed. The physician will know the best weight for a given height, age, and build and is the best source of advice for weight reduction.

Summary: The Role of Prevention

As important as it is to provide emergency treatment for the cardiac arrest victim, it is far more desirable to prevent cardiac arrest.[2,48] Risk factor modification has clearly been shown to save lives. The education of the layperson is essential in the effort to decrease mortality from CHD. Control of recognized risk factors depends on both the education and willingness of the public to understand and actively participate in changing to a healthier lifestyle. Evidence now exists that communitywide campaigns can be effective in reducing cardiovascular risks.

Educational efforts must also be directed toward overcoming patients' intrinsic denial of early evidence of cardiac disease and encouraging rapid entry into the EMS system when symptoms of CHD develop.

References

1. *Heart and Stroke Facts.* Dallas, Tex: American Heart Association; 1992.
2. Grundy SM, Greenland P, Herd A, et al. Cardiovascular and risk factor evaluation of healthy American adults: a statement for physicians by an Ad Hoc Committee appointed by the Steering Committee, American Heart Association. *Circulation.* 1987;75:1340A-1362A.
3. Gordon T, Kannel WB. Premature mortality from coronary heart disease: the Framingham Study. *JAMA.* 1971;215: 1617-1625.
4. Gordon T, Kannel WB. Multiple risk functions for predicting coronary heart disease: the concept, accuracy, and application. *Am Heart J.* 1982;103:1031-1039.
5. Gordon T, Kannel WB, McGee D, Dawber TR. Death and coronary attacks in men after giving up cigarette smoking: a report from the Framingham Study. *Lancet.* 1974;2: 1345-1348.
6. Wilhelmsson C, Vedin JA, Elmfeldt D, Tibblin G, Wilhelmsen L. Smoking and myocardial infarction. *Lancet.* 1975; 1:415-420.
7. Sparrow D, Dawber TR. The influence of cigarette smoking on prognosis after first myocardial infarction: a report from the Framingham Study. *J Chronic Dis.* 1978;31:425-432.
8. Castelli WP. Epidemiology of coronary heart disease: the Framingham Study. *Am J Med.* 1984;76(suppl 2A):4-12.
9. Kristein MM. 40 years of US cigarette smoking and heart disease and cancer mortality rates. *J Chronic Dis.* 1984;37: 317-323.
10. Ockene JK, Kuller LH, Svendsen KH, Meilahn E. The relationship of smoking cessation to coronary heart disease and lung cancer in the Multiple Risk Factor Intervention Trial (MRFIT). *Am J Public Health.* 1990;80:954-958.
11. Wells A. An estimate of adult mortality in the United States from passive smoking: a response to criticism. *Environ Int.* 1990;16:187-193.
12. Glantz SA, Parmley WW. Passive smoking and heart disease: epidemiology, physiology, and biochemistry. *Circulation.* 1991;83:1-12.
13. World Health Organisation European Collaborative Group. European collaborative trial of multifactorial prevention of coronary heart disease: final report on the 6-year results. *Lancet.* 1986;1:869-872.
14. Multiple Risk Factor Intervention Trial Research Group. Multiple risk factor intervention trial: risk factor changes and mortality results. *JAMA.* 1982;248:1465-1477.
15. Kannel WB, Neaton JD, Wentworth D, et al, for the MRFIT Research Group. Overall and coronary heart disease mortality rates in relation to major risk factors in 325,384 men screened for the MRFIT. *Am Heart J.* 1986;112:825-836.
16. Martin MJ, Hulley SB, Browner WS, Kuller LH, Wentworth D. Serum cholesterol, blood pressure, and mortality: implications from a cohort of 361,662 men. *Lancet.* 1986;2:933-936.
17. Multiple Risk Factor Intervention Trial Research Group. Coronary heart disease death, nonfatal acute myocardial infarction and other clinical outcomes in the Multiple Risk Factor Intervention Trial. *Am J Cardiol.* 1986;58:1-13.
18. The Pooling Project Research Group. Relationship of blood pressure, serum cholesterol, smoking habit, relative weight and ECG abnormalities to incidence of major coronary events: final report of the pooling project. *J Chronic Dis.* 1978;31:201-306.
19. Christakis G, Rinzler SH, Archer M, et al. The anti-coronary club: a dietary approach to the prevention of coronary heart disease — a seven-year report. *Am J Public Health Nations Health.* 1966; 56:299-314.
20. Christakis G, Rinzler SH, Archer M, Kraus A. Effect of the Anti-Coronary Club program on coronary heart disease risk-factor status. *JAMA.* 1966;198:597-604.
21. Miettinen M, Turpeinen O, Karvonen MJ, Elosuo R, Paavilainen E. Effect of cholesterol-lowering diet on mortality from coronary heart-disease and other causes: a twelve-year clinical trial in men and women. *Lancet.* 1972;2:835-838.
22. Dayton S, Pearce ML, Hashimoto S, Dixon WJ, Tomiyasu U. A controlled clinical trial of a diet high in unsaturated fat in preventing complications of atherosclerosis. *Circulation.* 1969;40(suppl 2):II-1-II-63.
23. Stamler J. Acute myocardial infarction: progress in primary prevention. *Br Heart J.* 1971;33(suppl):145-164.
24. Stamler J, Dyer AR, Shekelle RB, Neaton J, Stamler R. Relationship of baseline major risk factors to coronary and all-cause mortality, and to longevity: findings from long-term follow-up of Chicago cohorts. *Cardiology.* 1993;82:191-222.
25. *The Health Consequences of Smoking: Cardiovascular Disease: A Report of the Surgeon General.* Washington, DC: Office on Smoking and Health; 1983:127-129. US Dept of Health and Human Services publication 84-50204.
26. *The Health Consequences of Smoking for Women: A Report of the Surgeon General.* US Dept of Health and Human Services, Public Health Service, Office on Smoking and Health, 1980.
27. *Heart and Stroke Facts: 1994 Statistical Supplement.* Dallas, Tex: American Heart Association; 1993.
28. Miller WW. Preventive cardiology for coronary artery disease. *Prim Care.* 1985;12:15-38.

29. Goldstein JL, Brown MS. Familial hypercholesterolemia. In: Stanbury JB, Wyngarden JB, Fredrickson DS, Goldstein JL, Brown MS, eds. *The Metabolic Basis of Inherited Disease*. 5th ed. New York, NY: McGraw-Hill Book Co; 1983;672-713.

30. Stamler J, Wentworth D, Neaton JD. Is relationship between serum cholesterol and risk of premature death from coronary heart disease continuous and graded? Findings in 356,222 primary screenees of the Multiple Risk Factor Intervention Trial (MRFIT). *JAMA*. 1986;256:2823-2828.

31. The Lipid Research Clinics Coronary Primary Prevention Trial results, I: reduction in incidence of coronary heart disease. *JAMA*. 1984;251:351-364.

32. The Lipid Research Clinics Coronary Primary Prevention Trial results, II: the relationship of reduction in incidence of coronary heart disease to cholesterol lowering. *JAMA*. 1984;251:365-374.

33. *Diet in the Healthy Child*. Dallas, Tex: American Heart Association; 1983.

34. Morris JN, Heady JA, Raffle PAB, Roberts CG, Parks JW. Coronary heart disease and physical activity of work. *Lancet*. 1953;2:1053-1057; 1111-1120.

35. Paffenbarger RS, Hale WE. Work activity and coronary heart mortality. *N Engl J Med*. 1975;292:545-550.

36. Powell KE, Thompson PD, Caspersen CJ, Kendrick JS. Physical activity and the incidence of coronary heart disease. *Annu Rev Public Health*. 1987;8:253-287.

37. Oberman A. Exercise and the primary prevention of cardiovascular disease. *Am J Cardiol*. 1985;55:10D-20D.

38. Shephard RJ. Exercise in coronary heart disease. *Sports Med*. 1986;3:26-49.

39. Berlin JA, Colditz GA. A meta-analysis of physical activity in the prevention of coronary heart disease. *Am J Epidemiol*. 1990;132:612-628.

40. Stamler R, Stamler J, Lindberg HA, et al. Asymptomatic hyperglycemia and coronary heart disease in middle-aged men in two employed populations in Chicago. *J Chronic Dis*. 1979;32:805-815.

41. Ashley FW Jr, Kannel WB. Relation of weight change to changes in atherogenic traits: the Framingham Study. *J Chronic Dis*. 1974;27:103-114.

42. National Institutes of Health Consensus Development Panel on the Health Implications of Obesity. Health implications of obesity. *Ann Intern Med*. 1985;103:147-151.

43. Barrett-Connor EL. Obesity, atherosclerosis, and coronary artery disease. *Ann Intern Med*. 1985;103:1010-1019.

44. Hubert HB. The importance of obesity in the development of coronary risk factors and disease: the epidemiologic evidence. *Annu Rev Public Health*. 1986;7:493-502.

45. Hubert HB, Feinleib M, McNamara PM, Castelli WP. Obesity as an independent risk factor for cardiovascular disease: a 26-year follow-up of participants in the Framingham Heart Study. *Circulation*. 1983;678:968-977.

46. Manson JE, Colditz GA, Stampfer MJ, et al. A prospective study of obesity and risk of coronary heart disease in women. *N Engl J Med*. 1990;322:882-889.

47. Despres JP, Moorjani S, Lupien PJ, Tremblay A, Nadeau A, Bouchard C. Regional distribution of body fat, plasma lipoproteins, and cardiovascular disease. *Arteriosclerosis*. 1990;10:497-511.

48. Guidelines for cardiopulmonary resuscitation and emergency cardiac care, I: introduction. *JAMA*. 1992;268:2172-2183.

BLS is the phase of ECC that (1) prevents respiratory or cardiac arrest or insufficiency through prompt recognition and intervention or (2) supports the ventilation and circulation of a victim of cardiac arrest with CPR.[1] The major objective of performing rescue breathing or CPR is to provide oxygen to the brain and heart until appropriate, definitive medical treatment can restore normal heart and ventilatory action. The prompt administration of BLS is the key to success. In respiratory arrest, the survival rate may be very high if airway control and rescue breathing are started promptly.[1] For cardiac arrest the highest hospital discharge rate has been achieved in patients in whom BLS was initiated within 4 minutes of arrest and ACLS within 8 minutes.[2] For victims of sudden respiratory or cardiac arrest, early bystander BLS and a fast emergency medical services (EMS) response are essential in improving survival rates[3-5] and good neurological recovery rates.[6,7]

BLS education includes the teaching of primary and secondary prevention of respiratory and cardiac arrest. During the last 20 years the AHA has stressed that it is possible to prevent and control coronary heart disease by prudent heart living and risk factor modification.[8] The earlier this information is transmitted to the community, the stronger its impact on mortality and morbidity. Recent studies suggest that even school children can learn and implement heart-healthy living.

Training in CPR also includes information on danger signals, actions for survival, and entry into the EMS system to help prevent sudden death following myocardial infarction.

Citizen Response to Cardiopulmonary Emergencies

Previous guidelines have called for a single rescuer who is alone to perform CPR for 1 minute and then activate the EMS system.[9] Recent studies confirming the importance of early defibrillation have demonstrated a need to change this recommendation.[9]

The majority of sudden, adult, nontraumatic cardiac arrests are due to ventricular fibrillation (VF).[10] For these victims early defibrillation coupled with early bystander CPR maximizes the chance of survival.[11,12]

The time from collapse to defibrillation is critical. Most survivors of VF receive early defibrillation.[11,13] The beneficial effect of early defibrillation has been documented in part from improved survival rates in communities that have initiated an emergency medical technician-defibrillation (EMT-D) program.[14-18]

The window of opportunity for survival from sudden cardiac death is very narrow.[19] Anecdotal evidence suggests that trained lone rescuers often perform CPR for much longer than 1 minute, thereby delaying activation of the EMS system and the arrival of a defibrillator. In addition, witnesses of a collapse may call neighbors, relatives, or family physicians before activating the EMS system, further delaying defibrillation and decreasing the opportunity for survival from sudden cardiac death.[20,21]

A well-organized EMS system that can be accessed quickly through 911 (or another easily remembered telephone number) can often deliver early BLS, early defibrillation, and early advanced care. Such EMS systems offer the best chance for survival from sudden cardiac death[22] (Table 1).

Successful resuscitation has been observed in up to 61% of selected subgroups of out-of-hospital cardiac arrest victims when layperson CPR and an effective emergency response system capable of providing ACLS have been available within the community.[21] Thus, there are two indispensable links in the chain-of-survival approach to out-of-hospital cardiac arrest:

- Layperson education and training in CPR
- A mobile ECC capability that can make defibrillation available within minutes

Table 1. Relation of Survival Rates From Cardiac Arrest (Ventricular Fibrillation) to Promptness of CPR and ACLS.

Time to CPR (min)	Time to ACLS (min)	Survival rate (%)
0–4	0–8	43
0–4	16+	10
8–12	8–16	6
8–12	16+	0
12+	12+	0

From Eisenberg et al.[2] Reproduced with permission.

In every arrest, time is critical. There is usually enough oxygen in the lungs and bloodstream to support life for a few minutes. When breathing stops first, the heart will continue to pump blood for several minutes. Existing oxygen in the victim's lungs will continue to be circulated through the bloodstream to the brain and other vital organs. When the heart stops, however, the oxygen in the lungs and bloodstream is not circulated to the vital organs.

The victim whose circulation and breathing have been interrupted for less than 4 minutes has an excellent chance for full recovery if CPR is administered rapidly and followed by ACLS within the next 4 minutes (Table 1 and Fig 1). In the period from 4 to 6 minutes brain damage may occur. After 6 minutes brain damage will almost always occur.

For these reasons it is critically important for the nearest person to

- Recognize the need for immediate action. *Phone first!* Activate the EMS system.
- Perform the steps of CPR effectively.

Both trained and untrained bystanders should be instructed to call 911 or local emergency telephone numbers as soon as they have determined that an adult victim is unresponsive. If two bystanders are present, one should determine unresponsiveness and activate the EMS system and the other should begin

Sudden Cardiac Death

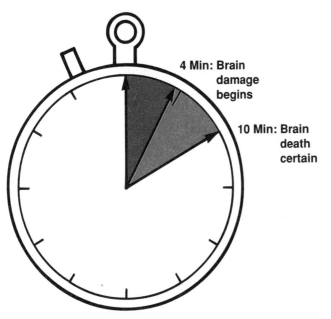

4 Min: Brain damage begins

10 Min: Brain death certain

Fig 1. Time is critical in starting CPR.

CPR. Emergency medical dispatchers must determine that the victim is unresponsive or that CPR is in progress in order to dispatch the appropriate rescue personnel and equipment. Emergency medical dispatchers have been identified as a vital part of the EMS system. In 1989 the National Association of EMS Physicians stated that "prearrival instructions are a mandatory function of each emergency medical dispatcher in a medical dispatch center" and "standard medically approved telephone instructions by trained [dispatchers] are safe to give and in many instances are a moral necessity."[23] If the rescuer does not know how to perform CPR or does not remember what steps to take, the dispatcher can instruct the rescuer in emergency measures, including CPR. Several studies have confirmed that dispatch-assisted CPR is practical and effective and can increase the likelihood that CPR will be performed.[24-26] Since telephone prearrival instructions must be based on the most accurate assessment of the patient's condition by the dispatcher, accurate written protocols must be used by dispatchers so that all necessary assessment information is obtained and concise, accurate instructions are provided.[27]

A potential concern about activating the EMS system before full assessment (by the single trained rescuer) is the delay incurred in treatment of primary respiratory arrest or an obstructed airway. In many situations that involve primary respiratory compromise — such as asphyxiation, drowning, strangulation, and respiratory arrest due to seizures, drug overdoses, or obstructed airway — airway opening and rescue breathing, not chest compression or defibrillation, are indicated. However, even trained rescuers may be unable to distinguish between primary cardiac arrest and a collapse secondary to airway and breathing problems. Hence, activating the EMS system immediately after determining unresponsiveness is still preferred in these victims.

When the emergency involves an infant (aged less than 1 year) or child (aged 1 to 8 years) instead of an adult, airway obstruction or respiratory arrest is far more likely to be present than cardiac arrest or VF.[28] In such situations CPR including rescue breathing is essential and should be done immediately.[9] After 1 minute of CPR, the lone rescuer should activate the EMS system. If either a conscious adult or child has an obstructed airway and the trained rescuer knows and can perform the proper technique, the obstructed airway maneuver should be attempted before activating the EMS system.[9]

Indications for BLS

Respiratory Arrest

When respiratory arrest occurs, the heart can continue to pump blood for several minutes, and oxygen will continue to circulate to the brain and other vital organs.[29] Persons with respiratory arrest commonly have a pulse. Early intervention for victims in whom respirations have stopped or the airway is obstructed may prevent cardiac arrest. Respiratory arrest can result from drowning, stroke, foreign-body airway obstruction, smoke inhalation, inflammation of the epiglottis (epiglottitis), drug overdose, electrocution, suffocation, injuries, or unconsciousness of any cause that leads to airway obstruction. Establishing a patent airway and delivering rescue breathing can save many lives in persons with inadequate respirations.

Cardiac Arrest

In cardiac arrest, circulation ceases and vital organs are deprived of oxygen. Ineffective "gasping" breathing efforts ("agonal" respirations) may occur early in cardiac arrest and should not be confused with effective respirations. If the victim has effective respirations, almost certainly the circulation is adequate and cardiac arrest is unlikely.

The Sequence of BLS: Assessment, EMS Activation, and the ABCs of CPR

The assessment phases of BLS are crucial. No victim should undergo CPR until the need for resuscitation has been established by the appropriate assessment.

Each of the ABCs of CPR — **A**irway, **B**reathing, and **C**irculation — begins with an assessment phase: determine unresponsiveness, determine breathlessness, and determine pulselessness. Assessment also involves a more subtle, constant process of observing and interacting with the victim. If unresponsiveness is established, the EMS system should be activated immediately.

Activate EMS

Assessment: Determine Unresponsiveness

The rescuer arriving at the side of the collapsed victim must quickly assess any injury and determine whether the person is responsive (Fig 2, top). The rescuer should tap or gently shake the victim and shout, "Are you OK?" If the victim does not respond, the EMS system should be promptly activated. If the victim has sustained trauma to the head and neck or trauma is suspected, the rescuer should move the victim only if absolutely necessary. Improper movement may cause paralysis in the victim with a spinal cord injury.

Activate the EMS System

The EMS system is activated by calling the local emergency telephone number (911, if available; Fig 2, bottom). This number should be widely publicized in each community. The person who calls the EMS system should be prepared to give the following information calmly[30]:

1. The location of the emergency (with names of cross streets or roads, if possible)
2. The telephone number from which the call is made
3. What happened — heart attack, auto accident, etc
4. How many people need help
5. Condition of the victim(s)
6. What aid is being given to the victim(s)
7. Any other information requested

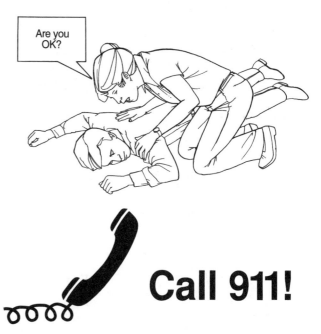

Fig 2. Initial steps of cardiopulmonary resuscitation. Top, Determine unresponsiveness; bottom, activate the emergency medical services system.

To ensure that EMS personnel have no more questions, the caller should hang up only when told to do so by the operator/dispatcher. The emergency medical dispatcher may (if so trained) give the caller instructions on how to initiate CPR. The caller should follow these instructions until skilled help arrives.

Airway

When the victim is unresponsive, the rescuer must determine if the victim is breathing. This assessment requires that the victim be positioned properly with the airway opened.

Position the Victim

For CPR to be effective, the victim must be supine and on a firm, flat surface. Blood flow to the brain may be compromised if the head is higher than the feet. Airway management and rescue breathing are also more easily achieved with the patient supine. It is imperative that the unconscious victim be positioned as quickly as possible. If the victim is lying face down, the rescuer must roll the victim as a unit ("log roll") so that the head, shoulders, and torso move simultaneously without twisting (Fig 3). Particular caution must be exercised if neck or back injury is suspected.

To position the victim who is lying down, the following sequence may be used:

- Kneel beside the victim at a distance approximately equal to the width of the victim's body and at the level of the victim's shoulders. This permits sufficient space to roll the victim while the neck is supported.

- Move the victim's arm closer to you so that it is raised above the victim's head.
- Straighten the victim's legs if necessary. They should be straight or bent slightly at the knees.
- Place one hand behind the victim's head and neck for support (Fig 3).
- With the other hand grasp the victim under the arm to brace the shoulder and torso.
- Roll the victim toward you by pulling steadily and evenly at the shoulder while controlling the head and neck. The head and neck should remain in the same plane as the torso, and the body should be moved as a unit.

The nonbreathing victim should be supine with the arms alongside the body. The victim is now appropriately positioned for the next step in CPR.

Rescuer Position

The rescuer should be at the victim's side, positioned to easily perform both rescue breathing and chest compression.

Open the Airway

One of the most important actions for successful resuscitation is immediate opening of the airway. In the unresponsive victim muscle tone is often impaired, resulting in the obstruction of the pharynx by the base of the tongue and the soft tissues of the pharynx (Fig 4, top).[31-35] The tongue is the most common cause of airway obstruction in the unconscious victim. The tongue or the epiglottis[34] may create an obstruction

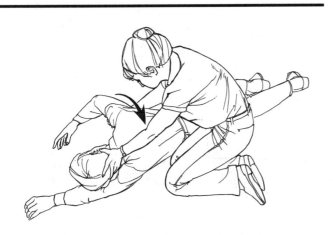

Fig 3. Positioning the victim. Victim must be supine and on a firm, flat surface.

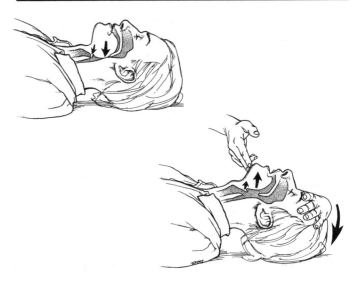

Fig 4. Opening the airway. Top, Airway obstruction produced by tongue and epiglottis; bottom, relief by head tilt–chin lift.

when negative pressure produced by inspiratory effort causes them to occlude the entrance to the trachea. Since the tongue is attached to the lower jaw, moving the lower jaw forward will lift the tongue away from the back of the throat and open the airway.

The rescuer should use the head tilt–chin lift maneuver to open the airway (Fig 4, bottom). If foreign material or vomitus is visible in the mouth, it should be removed. Excessive time must not be taken. Liquids or semiliquids should be wiped out with the index and middle fingers covered by a piece of cloth; solid material should be extracted with a hooked index finger.

Head Tilt–Chin Lift Maneuver. To perform the head tilt–chin lift maneuver:

- Place one hand on the victim's forehead and apply firm, backward pressure to tilt the head back.
- Place the fingers of the other hand under the bony part of the chin.
- Lift the chin forward and support the jaw, helping to tilt the head back.

Precautions:

- The fingers must not press deeply into the soft tissue under the chin, which might obstruct the airway.
- The thumb should not be used for lifting the chin.
- The mouth should not be closed.

When mouth-to-nose ventilation is needed, the hand that is already on the chin can be used to close the mouth to allow for effective mouth-to-nose ventilation.[34] If the victim has loose dentures, head tilt–chin lift makes a mouth-to-mouth seal easier.[36] Dentures should be removed if they cannot be kept in place.

Jaw-Thrust Maneuver. This technique is recommended as an alternative method of opening the airway by healthcare providers.

- Grasp the angles of the victim's lower jaw and lift with both hands, one on each side, displacing the mandible forward while tilting the head backward[37] (Fig 5).
- If the lips close, retreat the lower lip with the thumb.
- If mouth-to-mouth breathing is necessary, close the nostrils by placing your cheek tightly against them.[37]

This technique is effective in opening the airway[38,39] but is fatiguing and technically difficult.[36]

The jaw-thrust technique without head tilt is the safest approach to opening the airway of the victim with suspected neck injury because it usually can be accomplished without extending the neck. The head should be carefully supported without tilting it backward or turning it from side to side. If jaw thrust alone is unsuccessful, the head should be tilted backward very slightly.

Background on Airway-Opening Techniques

In 1960 Elam et al[38] described the technique for head tilt–chin lift: "Mouth-to-mouth and mouth-to-nose methods of artificial respiration are simplified and made more effective if the patient's neck is extended by the procedure here described. With the patient in the supine or semilateral position, the rescuer uses one hand to tilt the patient's head as far back as possible. He uses his other hand to pull the patient's chin upward."

There was no suggestion that the hand lifting the neck was to remain there. After tilting of the head, that hand was removed and used to support the chin. In fact, neck lift may not be needed. Lifting the chin and tilting the head may open the airway and accomplish the result more easily. Again, in Ruben et al[34] head tilt–neck lift was used only in the initial maneuver for tilting the head backward, not for opening or maintaining the airway or for mouth-to-mouth rescue breathing. Greene et al[40] stated: "When hyperextension of the head (50°) was produced by lifting the chin as well as pushing backward at the vertex or frontal region, a wider air passage uniformly appeared."

Guildner[36] stated the adequacy of three techniques for opening an airway obstructed by the tongue. The effectiveness of neck lift, chin lift, and jaw thrust, when combined with head tilt, were compared. Results indicated that chin lift provided the most consistently adequate airway.

Loose dentures posed a serious problem in mouth-to-mouth rescue breathing. By supporting the lower jaw and bringing the teeth almost to occlusion, head tilt–chin lift maintains the position of loose dentures and makes a mouth-to-mouth seal easier and more effective.

These data were reevaluated for the 1992 guidelines, and the recommendation for using head tilt–chin lift was again endorsed.

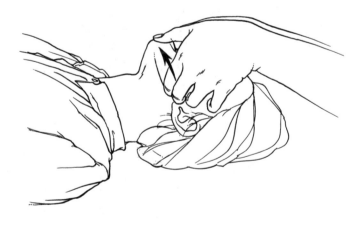

Fig 5. Jaw-thrust maneuver.

Breathing

BLS healthcare providers must be familiar with the use of a mask (or other barrier devices) with a one-way valve.

Assessment: Determine Breathlessness

To assess the presence or absence of spontaneous breathing:

- Place your ear over the victim's mouth and nose while maintaining an open airway (Fig 6).
- While observing the victim's chest
  — *Look* for the chest to rise and fall
  — *Listen* for air escaping during exhalation
  — *Feel* for the flow of air

If the chest does not rise and fall and no air is exhaled, the victim is breathless. This evaluation procedure should take only 3 to 5 seconds.

It should be stressed that although the rescuer may notice that the victim is making respiratory efforts, the airway may still be obstructed, and opening the airway may be all that is needed. In addition, reflex gasping respiratory efforts (agonal respirations) may occur early in the course of primary cardiac arrest and should not be mistaken for adequate breathing.

Recovery Position. If the victim is unresponsive, has no evidence of trauma, and is obviously breathing adequately, the rescuer should place the patient in the "recovery position" (Fig 7):

- Roll the victim onto his or her side so that the head, shoulders, and torso move simultaneously without twisting.
- If the victim has sustained trauma or trauma is suspected, the victim should **not** be moved.

In the recovery position, the airway is more likely to remain open, and unrecognized airway obstruction (by virtue of the tongue falling back) is less likely to occur. It is essential to continue close observation of the victim who has been placed in the recovery position until he or she becomes responsive or until skilled providers arrive to assume care of the victim. The recovery position may also be employed in victims who are successfully resuscitated. If continued observation and monitoring of such resuscitated victims has to be interrupted to perform another vital task and the victim is still supine, the victim should be placed in the recovery position.

Perform Rescue Breathing

Mouth to Mouth. Rescue breathing with the mouth-to-mouth technique is a quick, effective way to provide oxygen to the victim[41] (Fig 8). The rescuer's exhaled air contains enough oxygen to supply the victim's needs. Rescue breathing requires that the rescuer inflate the victim's lungs adequately with each breath.

- Keep the airway open by the head tilt–chin lift maneuver.

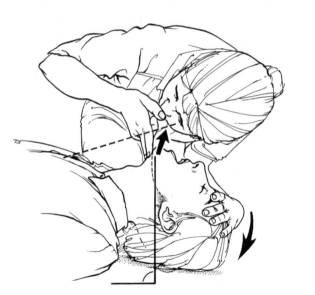

Fig 6. Determining breathlessness.

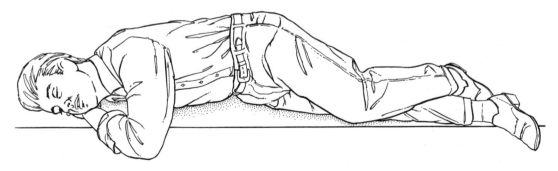

Fig 7. Placing the victim in the recovery position.

- Gently pinch the nose closed with your thumb and index finger (of the hand on the forehead), thereby preventing air from escaping through the victim's nose.
- Take a deep breath and seal your lips around the victim's mouth, creating an airtight seal.
- Then give two slow breaths.

Adequate time for the two breaths *(1½ to 2 seconds per breath)* should be allowed to provide good chest expansion and decrease the possibility of gastric distention. (Measurements of time "per breath" given here are indicative of the victim's inspiratory time.) The rescuer should take a breath after each ventilation, and each individual ventilation should be of sufficient volume to make the chest rise. In most adults, this volume will be 800 to 1200 mL (0.8 to 1.2 L).

Rescue breathing should be performed at a *rate of 10 to 12 breaths per minute.* Too great a volume of air and too fast an inspiratory flow rate are likely to cause pharyngeal pressures that exceed esophageal opening pressures, allowing air to enter the stomach and resulting in gastric distention.[42-44] Adequate ventilation is indicated by

- Observing the chest rise and fall
- Hearing and feeling the air escape during exhalation.

When possible the airway should be kept patent during exhalation to minimize gastric distention.

If attempts to ventilate the victim are unsuccessful, reposition the victim's head and reattempt rescue breathing. Improper chin and head positioning is the most common cause of difficulty with ventilation. If the victim cannot be ventilated after repositioning the head, proceed with foreign-body airway maneuvers (see "Foreign-Body Airway Obstruction Management").

Mouth to Nose. This technique is more effective in some cases than the mouth-to-mouth technique[45] (Fig 9). The mouth-to-nose technique is recommended when it is impossible to ventilate through the victim's mouth, the mouth cannot be opened (trismus), the mouth is seriously injured, or a tight mouth-to-mouth seal is difficult to achieve.

- Keep the victim's head tilted back with one hand on the forehead.
- Use the other hand to lift the victim's lower jaw (as in head tilt–chin lift) and close the mouth.
- Take a deep breath, seal your lips around the victim's nose, and blow.
- Then stop rescue breathing and allow the victim to exhale passively.

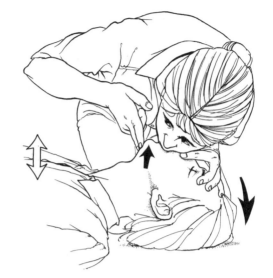

Fig 8. Mouth-to-mouth rescue breathing.

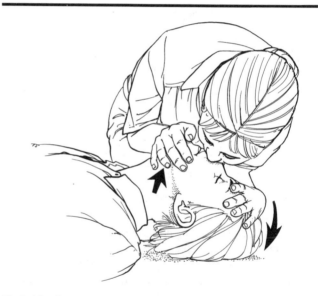

Fig 9. Mouth-to-nose breathing.

It may be necessary to open the victim's mouth intermittently or separate the lips with the thumb to allow air to be exhaled since nasal obstruction may be present during exhalation.[46]

Mouth to Stoma. Persons who have undergone a laryngectomy (surgical removal of the larynx) have a permanent opening that connects the trachea directly to the front of the neck.[47] When such a person requires rescue breathing, direct mouth-to-stoma ventilation should be performed (Figs 10 and 11).

- Make an airtight seal around the stoma and blow slowly until the chest rises.

- When rescue breathing is stopped, the victim exhales passively.

Other victims may have a temporary tracheostomy tube in the trachea. To ventilate such a person, the

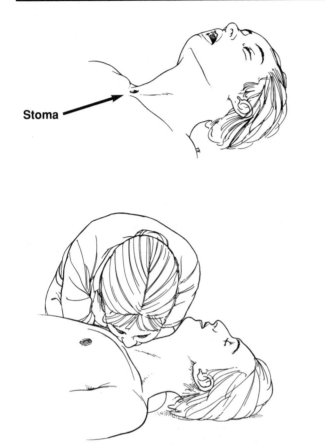

Stoma

Fig 10. Top, Anatomy of a permanent stoma. Bottom, Mouth-to-stoma rescue breathing. Adapted from *Cardiopulmonary Resuscitation.* Washington, DC: American Red Cross; 1987:16, 17.

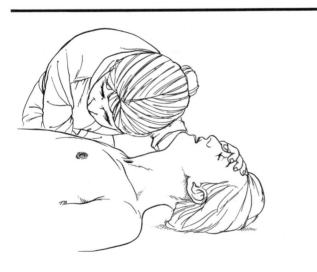

Fig 11. Assessing respirations at the stoma.

victim's mouth and nose usually must be sealed by the rescuer's hand or by a tightly fitting face mask to prevent leakage of air when the rescuer blows into the tracheostomy tube. This problem is alleviated when the tracheostomy tube has an inflated cuff. If unable to ventilate through a tracheostomy tube, the tube should be removed and ventilation attempted directly through the stoma.

Mouth to Barrier Device. Some rescuers may prefer to use a barrier device during mouth-to-mouth ventilation. Two broad categories of devices are available: masks and face shields. Most masks have a one-way valve so that exhaled air does not enter the rescuer's mouth. Many face shields have no exhalation valve, and often air leaks around the shield. Barrier devices should ideally have a low resistance to gas flow, or the user may tire from excessive respiratory effort. If rescue breathing is necessary, position the barrier device (face mask or face shield) over the victim's mouth and nose, ensuring an adequate air seal. Then initiate mouth-to–barrier device breathing using slow inspiratory breaths (1½ to 2 seconds).

Mouth-to-Mask Rescue Breathing. The mouth-to-mask breathing device includes a transparent mask with a one-way valve mouthpiece. The one-way valve directs the rescuer's breath into the victim's airway while diverting the victim's exhaled air away from the rescuer. Some devices have an oxygen adaptor that permits the administration of supplemental oxygen.

Mouth-to-mask is a reliable form of ventilation since it allows the rescuer to use two hands to create a mask seal. The technique for use of the mouth-to-mask device:

- Place the mask around the patient's mouth and nose using the bridge of the nose as a guide for correct position. Positioning of the mask is critical because gaps between the mask and face will result in air leakage.
- Seal the mask by placing the heel and thumb of each hand along the border of the mask and compressing firmly to provide a tight seal around the margin of the mask.
- Place your remaining fingers along the boney margin of the jaw and lift the jaw while performing a head tilt (Fig 4, bottom).
- Give breaths in the same sequence and at the same rate as in rescue breathing, observing chest excursion.

Use of the mask during two-person CPR can be done in a variety of ways. Individual systems should determine what works best with their equipment and their people.

Cricoid Pressure. This technique consists of applying backward pressure on the cricoid cartilage to compress the esophagus against the cervical vertebra to prevent gastric insufflation and possible regurgitation.[48,49] Cricoid pressure has been effective in preventing regurgitation against esophageal pressure of up to 100 cm H_2O.[50] This technique should be used only by healthcare professionals in two-rescuer CPR. The procedure is simple but cannot be accomplished by a single rescuer.

Recommendations for Rescue Breathing

- Give two initial breaths of 1½ to 2 seconds each.
- For both one-rescuer and two-rescuer CPR, deliver 10 to 12 breaths per minute.
- In one-rescuer CPR, pause for ventilation after every 15 chest compressions.
- In two-rescuer CPR, pause for ventilation after every 5 chest compressions.

By giving the ventilations with a slow inspiratory flow rate and avoiding trapping of air in the lungs between breaths, the possibility of exceeding the esophageal opening pressure will be less. This technique should result in less gastric distention, regurgitation, and aspiration.

The 1½- to 2-second time period for ventilation is to deliver slow inspiratory breaths. Exhalation is a passive phenomenon and occurs primarily during chest compressions if CPR is being performed.

Circulation

Assessment: Determine Pulselessness

Cardiac arrest is recognized by pulselessness in the large arteries of the unconscious victim (Fig 12).

- Check the pulse at the carotid artery; this should take no more than 5 to 10 seconds.
- The carotid artery is the most accessible, reliable, and easily learned location for checking the pulse in adults and children. This artery lies in a groove created by the trachea and the large strap muscles of the neck.
- While maintaining head tilt with one hand on the forehead, locate the victim's larynx with two or three fingers of the other hand.
- Place these fingers into the groove between the trachea and the muscles at the side of the neck, where the carotid pulse can be felt (Fig 12, bottom).

The pulse area must be pressed gently to avoid compressing the artery. This technique is more easily performed on the side nearer the rescuer. Simulta-

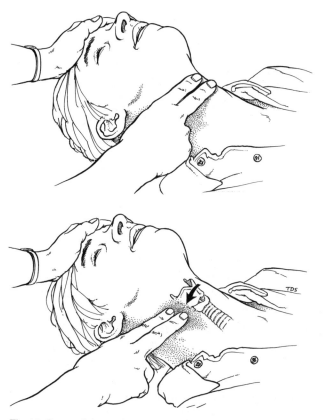

Fig 12. Determining pulselessness. Locate the larynx while maintaining the head-tilt position (top). Slide the fingers into the groove between the trachea and the muscles at the side of the neck where the carotid pulse can be felt (bottom).

neous palpation of both carotid arteries should never be done since it can obstruct blood flow to the brain.

The pulse in the carotid artery may persist even when more peripheral pulses (eg, radial) are no longer palpable. Determining pulselessness using the femoral artery pulse is also acceptable for healthcare professionals. However, this pulse is difficult to locate in a fully clothed patient.

The victim's condition must be properly assessed since performing chest compressions on an adult who has a pulse may result in serious medical complications.

If There Is a Pulse. Locating and palpating a pulse will take 5 to 10 seconds. It takes time to find the correct location, and the pulse may be slow, irregular, or very weak and rapid.

If a pulse is present but there is no breathing, rescue breathing should be initiated at a rate of 10 to 12 times per minute, or once every 5 to 6 seconds (after the initial two breaths of 1½ to 2 seconds each).

If There Is No Pulse. If no pulse is palpated, the victim is in cardiac arrest. At this point, if the EMS system has not already been activated, it should be, and chest compressions should be begun.

Chest Compressions

Cardiac arrest is recognized by pulselessness in the large arteries of the unconscious, breathless victim. As mentioned earlier, agonal gasping breathing may occur during the first several minutes of cardiac arrest and should not be mistaken for adequate respirations. If a victim has adequate ventilations, almost certainly the circulation is also adequate and cardiac arrest is unlikely. For the victim of cardiac arrest all the ABCs of CPR are required in rapid succession to optimize the chances for survival.

The chest compression technique consists of serial, rhythmic applications of pressure over the lower half of the sternum[51] (Fig 13). These compressions provide circulation as a result of a generalized increase in intrathoracic pressure or direct compression of the heart.[52,53] Blood circulated to the lungs by chest compressions will likely receive enough oxygen to maintain life when the compressions are accompanied by properly performed rescue breathing.[54]

The patient must be in the horizontal, supine position during chest compressions. Even with properly performed compressions, blood flow to the brain is reduced. Whenever the head is elevated above the heart, blood flow to the brain is further reduced or even eliminated. If the victim is in bed, a board, preferably the full width of the bed, should be placed under the patient's back.

Proper Hand Position. Proper hand placement is established by identifying the lower half of the sternum. The guidelines below may be used, or the rescuer may choose alternative techniques to identify the lower sternum.

- With your hand locate the lower margin of the victim's rib cage on the side next to the rescuer.
- Move the fingers up the rib cage to the notch where the ribs meet the sternum in the center of the lower part of the chest.
- Place the heel of one hand on the lower half of the sternum, and place the other hand on top of the hand on the sternum so that the hands are parallel (Fig 13, left). The long axis of the heel of the rescuer's hand should be placed on the long axis of the sternum. This will keep the main force of compression on the sternum and decrease the chance of rib fracture.
- The fingers may be either extended or interlaced but should be kept off the chest.

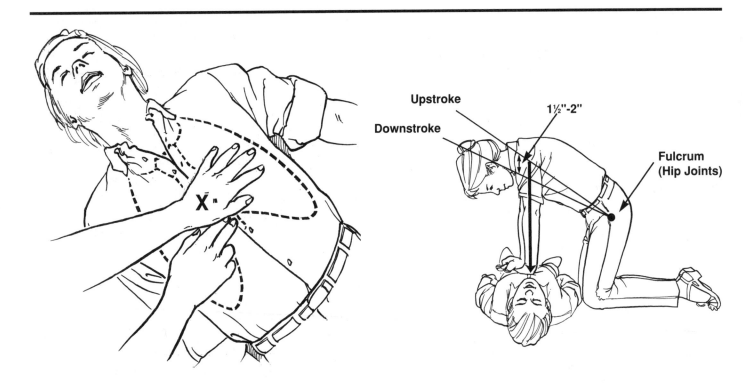

Fig 13. Chest compression. Left, Locating the correct hand position on the lower half of the sternum; right, proper position of the rescuer, with shoulders directly over the victim's sternum and elbows locked. Adapted from *Cardiopulmonary Resuscitation*. Washington, DC: American National Red Cross; 1981:25.

- An acceptable alternative hand position is to grasp the wrist of the hand on the chest with the hand that has been locating the lower end of the sternum. This technique is helpful for rescuers with arthritic hands and wrists.

Proper Compression Techniques. Effective compression is accomplished by attention to the following guidelines (Fig 13, right):

- Your elbows should preferably be locked into position, your arms straightened, and your shoulders positioned directly over the hands so that the thrust for each chest compression is straight down on the sternum. If the thrust is not in a straight downward direction, the torso has a tendency to roll. Part of the downward force is displaced, and the chest compression may be less effective.
- To achieve the most pressure with the least effort, lean forward until your shoulders are directly over your outstretched hands (ie, lean forward until the body reaches natural imbalance — a point at which there would be a sensation of falling forward if the hands and arms were not providing support). The weight of your back creates the necessary pressure that makes compressions easier on the arms and shoulders. Natural body weight falling forward provides the force to depress the sternum.
- The sternum should be depressed approximately 1½ to 2 inches (3.8 to 5.1 cm) for the normal-sized adult. Rarely, in very slight persons lesser degrees of compression may be enough to generate a palpable carotid or femoral pulse. In some persons 1½ to 2 inches of sternal compression may be inadequate and a slightly greater degree of chest compression may be needed to generate an adequate carotid or femoral pulse. Ideally, optimal sternal compression is best gauged by using the compression force that generates a palpable carotid or femoral pulse. However, simultaneous chest compression and a pulse palpation can be implemented only by two rescuers. The single rescuer should follow the sternal compression guideline of 1½ to 2 inches.
- Release chest compression pressure between each compression to allow blood to flow into the chest and heart. The pressure must be released and the chest allowed to return to its normal position after each compression. Arterial pressure during chest compression is maximal when the duration of compression is 50% of the compression-release cycle.[36] Hence, rescuers should be encouraged to maintain prolonged

Physiology of Circulation

Closed-chest cardiac massage was described in 1960.[51] Soon after, this technique was accepted by healthcare professionals and later by laypersons and became known as "standard" or "conventional" CPR.

It was believed that chest compression resulted in direct compression of the heart between the sternum and the spine, causing an increase in pressure within the ventricles and a closure of the valves (mitral and tricuspid). This pressure was thought to cause blood to move into the pulmonary artery (to the lungs) and the aorta (blood flow to the organs).

This "cardiac pump theory"[55] is supported by recent studies that demonstrated that stroke volume and coronary blood flow are higher with high-impulse (moderate to high force and brief duration) chest compressions at high rates[52] and that the timing of valve opening and closure occurs as initially hypothesized.[56] Mitral valve closure and cardiac chamber compression during chest compression have also been reported in some but not all transthoracic human echocardiographic studies.[57,58]

This conventional theory of blood flow during CPR has been challenged by several workers who have advanced the "thoracic pump mechanism."[53,59,60] According to this theory, chest compression produces a rise in intrathoracic pressure that is transmitted equally to all intrathoracic vascular structures. Because arteries resist collapse, there is nearly full transmission of pressure from intrathoracic to extrathoracic arteries. Competent venous valves and venous collapse prevent full transmission of pressure to extrathoracic veins. An extrathoracic arteriovenous pressure gradient is produced, which causes blood to flow. This thoracic pump theory is supported by the following observations:

- In patients with flail chests undergoing CPR, the arterial pressure does not increase during chest compressions unless the chest is stabilized with a belt, which allows an increase in intrathoracic pressure.[53]
- Some patients with witnessed ventricular fibrillation and cardiac arrest who are asked to cough vigorously before loss of consciousness are able to remain conscious, and the systolic arterial pressure during coughing is higher than 100 mm Hg. This significant increase in intrathoracic pressure provides blood flow to the brain and heart.[61] The increase in intrathoracic pressure during coughing results from the contraction of the diaphragm and intercostal and abdominal muscles against a closed glottis.
- Similar to the intravascular pressures observed in animals (where the thoracic pump concept has been confirmed), intravascular pressure recordings in patients undergoing CPR have demonstrated equivalent right and left heart pressures and a negative jugular venous to right heart pressure difference during chest compression.[62]

Mitral valve closure during chest compression was thought to be one of the hallmarks of the cardiac pump theory. Detailed echocardiography in animals has demonstrated, however, that mitral valve closure during chest compression may occur whether blood flow during CPR is a consequence of either the cardiac pump or the thoracic pump. Thus mitral valve motion cannot be used to index the mechanism of flow during CPR.[63,64]

It is possible that both mechanisms for blood flow play a role during chest compression in man. Which is predominant in a particular victim may depend on several factors, including the size of the heart, ventrodorsal chest diameter, compliance of the chest wall, magnitude of chest compressions, and perhaps other unknown factors.

chest compression. This is more easily achieved at faster chest compression rates (80 to 100 per minute).

- Do not lift the hands from the chest or change position, or correct hand position may be lost.

Bouncing compressions, jerky movements, improper hand position, and leaning on the chest can decrease the effectiveness of resuscitation and are more likely to cause injuries.

Rescue breathing and chest compression must be combined for effective resuscitation of the victim of cardiopulmonary arrest. *The chest compression rate should be a minimum of 80 to 100 per minute if possible,* and duration of chest compression should be 50% of the compression-release cycle.

Recommendations for Chest Compression.

- The chest compression rate should be a minimum of 80 per minute and up to 100 per minute if possible.

This rate is consistent with both the cardiac pump and the thoracic pump theories of blood flow. If direct compression of the heart is operative, it is clear that a faster rate will increase blood flow. If the increase in intrathoracic pressure is the mechanism of blood flow during CPR, faster compression rates make it easier to maintain chest compression for a duration of 50% of cycle time and thereby increase flow to the brain and the heart.

Infrequently the rescuer may encounter a victim with unusual chest wall anatomy, eg, a chest with a markedly depressed sternum or a patient who has had extensive chest wall reconstructive surgery. The physiology of blood flow during CPR suggests that in such victims chest compressions should be performed as described above with hand position approximated to the sternal-anterior chest anatomy.

During cardiac arrest, properly performed chest compressions can produce systolic arterial blood pressure peaks of 60 to 80 mm Hg, but diastolic blood pressure is low.[62] Mean blood pressure in the carotid artery seldom exceeds 40 mm Hg.[62] Cardiac output resulting from chest compressions is likely only one fourth to one third of normal but has not been well studied.[62] Vascular pressure during chest compression can be optimized by using the appropriate recommended chest compression force, prolonging chest compression duration, and maintaining a chest compression rate of 80 to 100 per minute.

Recently there has been important research in various new techniques to improve blood flow during

CPR: pneumatic vest CPR, interposed abdominal compression CPR (IAC-CPR), and active compression-decompression CPR (ACD-CPR). Evaluation of their use in humans has been limited, though initially promising. More information about survival rates, neurological outcome, and complications in patients is needed before changes in the techniques of CPR are recommended.

Airway-breathing-circulation (ABC) is the specific sequence used to initiate CPR. However, in the Netherlands, "CAB" is the common strategy for CPR implementation, with resuscitation outcomes similar to those reported for the ABCs in the United States. No human studies have compared the ABC technique of resuscitation with CAB. Hence a statement of relative efficacy cannot be made, and a change in present teaching is not warranted. Both techniques are effective.

Cough CPR

Self-induced CPR is possible. However, its use is limited to clinical situations in which the patient has a cardiac monitor, the arrest was recognized before loss of consciousness (usually within 10 to 15 seconds from the cardiac arrest), and the patient can cough forcefully.[61] The increase in intrathoracic pressure will generate blood flow to the brain to maintain consciousness for a prolonged period.[65]

CPR Performed by One Rescuer and by Two Rescuers

CPR Performed by One Trained Rescuer

One-rescuer CPR is effective in maintaining adequate circulation and ventilation but is more exhausting than two-rescuer CPR. When trained healthcare providers arrive at the scene of an emergency, they should proceed with two-rescuer CPR and ACLS, as appropriate.

Sequence for Adult One-Rescuer CPR

	Assessment: Determine unresponsiveness.
	• Tap or gently shake the victim and shout.
	• Activate the EMS system.
AIRWAY	• Position the victim.
	• Open the airway by the head tilt–chin lift maneuver.
BREATHING	**Assessment:** Determine breathlessness.
	• If the victim is unresponsive but obviously breathing and if there is no trauma, *place the victim in the recovery position* and maintain an open airway.
	• If the adult victim is unresponsive and not breathing, perform rescue breathing by giving two initial breaths.
	• If unable to give two breaths, reposition the head and attempt to ventilate again.
	• If still unsuccessful, perform the foreign-body airway obstruction sequence.
CIRCULATION	**Assessment:** Determine pulselessness.
	• If pulse is present and the victim is unresponsive, continue rescue breathing at 10 to 12 times per minute.
	• If pulse is absent, begin chest compression.
	— Perform 15 chest compressions at a rate of 80 to 100 per minute. Count "one and, two and, three and, four and, five and, six and, seven and, eight and, nine and, ten and, eleven and, twelve and, thirteen and, fourteen and, fifteen." (Any mnemonic that helps maintain the same compression rate is acceptable.)
	— Open the airway and deliver two slow rescue breaths (1½ to 2 seconds each).
	— Find the proper hand position and begin 15 more compressions at a rate of 80 to 100 per minute.
	— Perform four complete cycles of 15 compressions and two ventilations.

Reassessment

• After four cycles of compressions and ventilations (15:2 ratio), reevaluate the patient.
• Check for return of the carotid pulse (3 to 5 seconds).
• *If absent, resume CPR with chest compressions.*
• If a pulse is present, check breathing.
   — If present, closely monitor breathing and pulse.
   — If absent, perform rescue breathing at 10 to 12 times per minute and monitor pulse closely.
• If effective breathing is present for several minutes and the victim has to be left unattended to perform another vital task, place the victim in the recovery position.

If CPR is continued, stop and check for return of pulse and spontaneous breathing every few minutes. Do not interrupt CPR except in special circumstances.

Summary: The One-Rescuer Decision Tree

The one-rescuer CPR decision tree (Fig 14) is a review of all the steps for one-rescuer CPR for the unconscious adult victim.

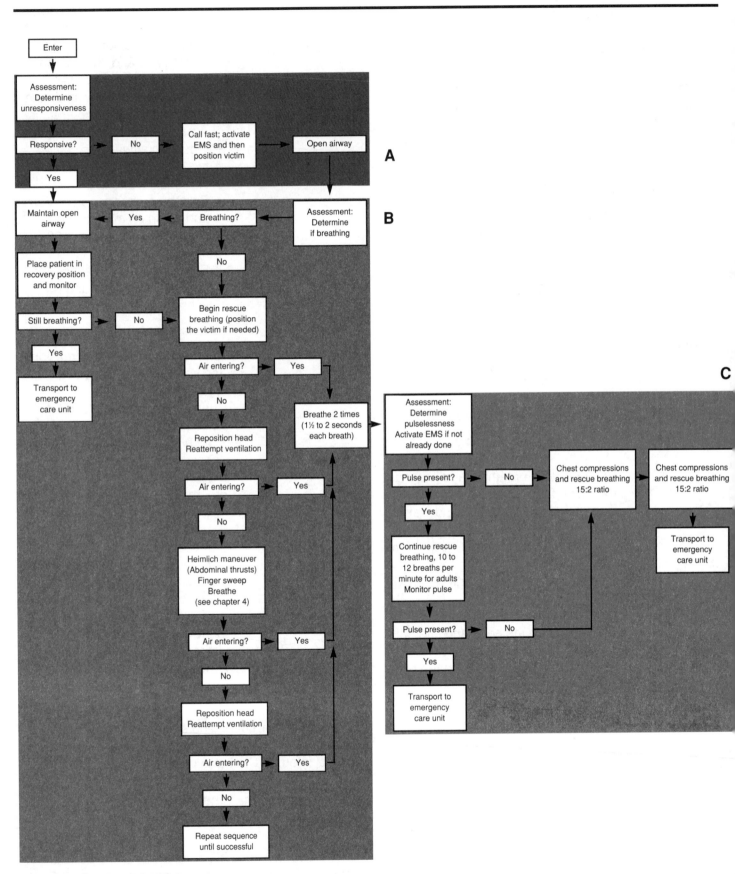

Fig 14. One-rescuer CPR decision tree.

One-Rescuer CPR With Entry of a Second Rescuer

When another rescuer is available at the scene, the second rescuer should activate the EMS system (if not done previously) and perform one-rescuer CPR when the first rescuer, who initiated CPR, becomes fatigued. This should be done with as little interruption as possible. When the second rescuer arrives, breathing and pulse should be reassessed before CPR is resumed. For example, the first rescuer completes a cycle of 15 chest compressions and gives 2 breaths. *If after a pulse check no pulse is present, the second rescuer resumes chest compressions and does not precede this with ventilation (since this has just occurred).* This approach to integration of the second rescuer is designed for simplicity.

CPR Performed by Two Rescuers

All healthcare providers should learn both the one-rescuer and the two-rescuer techniques. The latter is less fatiguing. In the two-rescuer technique for two healthcare providers, mouth-to-mask ventilation is an acceptable alternative to rescue breathing.

Advantages of Two-Rescuer CPR

Because artificial circulation must be combined with artificial ventilation, it is preferable to have two rescuers. One rescuer, positioned at the victim's side, performs chest compressions while the other rescuer, positioned at the victim's head, maintains an open airway and performs ventilations. The compression rate for two-rescuer CPR, as for one-rescuer CPR, is 80 to 100 per minute. The compression ventilation ratio is 5:1 with a pause for ventilation of 1½ to 2 seconds consisting primarily of inspiration. Exhalation occurs during chest compressions. When performed in two-rescuer CPR without interruptions, this rate yields approximately 60 chest compressions per minute and can maintain adequate blood flow and pressure, reduce rescuer fatigue, and provide for more ventilations. When the person doing chest compressions becomes fatigued, the rescuers should exchange positions as soon as possible.

Monitoring the Victim

The victim's condition must be monitored to assess the effectiveness of the rescue effort. The person ventilating the patient assumes the responsibility for monitoring pulse and breathing, which serves to

- Evaluate the effectiveness of compressions
- Determine if the victim resumes spontaneous circulation and breathing

To assess the effectiveness of the partner's chest compressions, the rescuer should check the pulse during the compressions. To determine if the victim has resumed spontaneous breathing and circulation, chest compressions must be stopped for 5 seconds at about the end of the first minute and every few minutes thereafter.

How an Untrained Lay Rescuer Can Help

An untrained lay rescuer can help a trained lay rescuer who is performing one-rescuer CPR by activating the appropriate emergency system or by assisting the trained rescuer as directed.

Explain CPR

If the single rescuer is exhausted, it may be best to have the novice help perform CPR briefly so that the initial rescuer can regain strength and resume CPR until help arrives. Since compressions are easier to learn by observation than rescue breathing is, tell the novice to watch what is being done and to copy the movements carefully. Tell the novice to watch how the chest is compressed:

- Point out the hand location on the victim's chest.
- Explain how to keep the arms straight and the shoulders over the victim's chest.

Novice Takes Over

The first rescuer should observe the novice's hands as the proper position is located.

- Alert the novice to be prepared to assume the same chest position as that of the first rescuer.
- Remind the novice that chest compressions should begin immediately and be continued without interruption.

As soon as the novice has begun compressions, the first rescuer should begin rescue breathing.

Monitor the Novice

While performing rescue breathing, the experienced rescuer must constantly monitor the novice's performance and make corrections in technique.

As soon as strength is regained, the experienced rescuer should resume one-person CPR unless the novice is performing adequate compressions.

Foreign-Body Airway Obstruction Management

Causes and Precautions

Upper airway obstruction can cause unconsciousness and cardiopulmonary arrest, but far more often unconsciousness and cardiopulmonary arrest cause upper airway obstruction.

An unconscious patient can develop airway obstruction when the tongue falls backward into the pharynx, obstructing the upper airway. Regurgitation of stomach contents into the pharynx, resulting in an obstructed airway, can occur during a cardiopulmonary arrest or during resuscitative attempts. Bleeding from head and facial injuries may also obstruct the upper airway, particularly if the patient is unconscious.

The National Safety Council[66] reported that foreign-body obstruction of the airway accounted for approximately 3900 deaths in 1989. Management of upper airway obstruction is taught within the context of BLS because of the associated ventilatory and circulatory problems if the victim becomes unconscious.

Foreign-body airway obstruction should be considered in any victim, especially a younger victim, who suddenly stops breathing, becomes cyanotic, and loses consciousness for no apparent reason. Foreign-body obstruction of the airway usually occurs during eating. In adults, meat is the most common cause of obstruction, although a variety of other foods and foreign bodies have been the cause of choking in children and some adults. Common factors associated with choking on food include large, poorly chewed pieces of food, elevated blood alcohol levels, and dentures. In restaurants this emergency has been mistaken for a heart attack, giving rise to the term "café coronary."[67]

People may help prevent foreign-body airway obstruction by

- Cutting food into small pieces and chewing slowly and thoroughly, especially if wearing dentures
- Avoiding laughing and talking during chewing and swallowing
- Avoiding excessive intake of alcohol
- Restricting children from walking, running, or playing when they have food in their mouths
- Keeping foreign objects (eg, marbles, beads, thumbtacks) away from infants and children
- Withholding peanuts, peanut butter, popcorn, hot dogs, and other foods that must be thoroughly chewed from children unable to do so.

Recognition of Foreign-Body Airway Obstruction

Because early recognition of airway obstruction is the key to successful outcome, it is important to distinguish this emergency from fainting, stroke, heart attack, epilepsy, drug overdose, or other conditions that cause sudden respiratory failure but are treated differently.

Foreign bodies may cause either partial or complete airway obstruction. With partial airway obstruction, the victim may be capable of either "good air exchange" or "poor air exchange." With good (adequate) air exchange, the victim remains conscious and can cough forcefully, although frequently there is wheezing between coughs. As long as good air exchange continues, the victim should be encouraged to continue spontaneous coughing and breathing efforts. At this point do *not* interfere with the victim's attempts to expel the foreign body, but stay with the victim and monitor these attempts. If partial airway obstruction persists, activate the EMS system.

Poor (inadequate) air exchange may occur initially, or good air exchange may progress to poor air exchange, as indicated by a weak, ineffective cough, high-pitched noise while inhaling, increased respiratory difficulty, and possibly cyanosis. A partial obstruction with poor air exchange should be treated as if it were a complete airway obstruction.

With complete airway obstruction the victim is unable to speak, breathe, or cough and may clutch the neck with the thumb and fingers (Fig 15). (The public should be encouraged to use this sign, the universal distress signal, when choking.) Ask the victim if he or she is choking. Movement of air will be absent if complete airway obstruction is present. Oxygen saturation in the blood will decrease rapidly because the obstructed airway prevents entry of air into the lungs, resulting in unconsciousness. Death will follow rapidly if prompt action is not taken.

Management of the Obstructed Airway

The Heimlich maneuver (subdiaphragmatic abdominal thrusts) is recommended for relieving foreign-body airway obstruction.[68] By elevating the diaphragm, the Heimlich maneuver can force air from the lungs to create an artificial cough intended to expel a foreign body obstructing the airway.[69-75] Each individual thrust should be administered with the intent of relieving the obstruction. It may be necessary to repeat the thrust multiple times during each sequence to clear the airway.

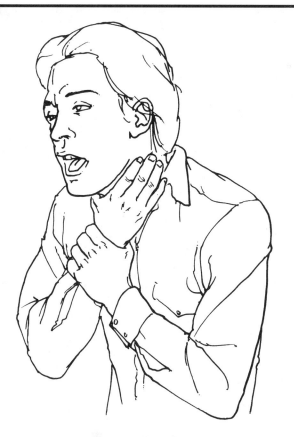

Fig 15. Universal distress signal for foreign-body airway obstructions.

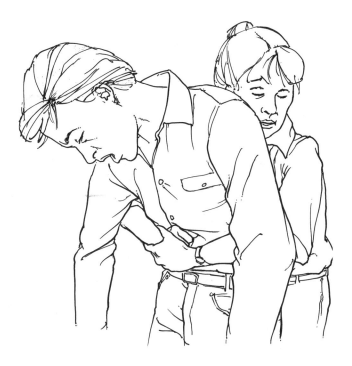

Fig 16. Heimlich maneuver administered to conscious victim of foreign-body airway obstruction who is sitting or standing.

An important consideration during the maneuver is possible damage to internal organs, such as rupture or laceration of abdominal or thoracic viscera.[76,77] To minimize this possibility, the rescuer's hands should never be placed on the xiphoid process of the sternum or on the lower margins of the rib cage. They should be below this area but above the navel and in the midline.

Regurgitation may occur as a result of abdominal thrusts. Training and proper performance should minimize these problems.

Heimlich Maneuver With Victim Standing or Sitting

The rescuer should stand behind the victim, wrap his or her arms around the victim's waist, and proceed as follows (Fig 16):

- Make a fist with one hand.
- Place the thumb side of the fist against the victim's abdomen, in the midline slightly above the navel and well below the tip of the xiphoid process.
- Grasp the fist with the other hand and press the fist into the victim's abdomen with a quick upward thrust.

- Repeat the thrusts and continue until the object is expelled from the airway or the patient becomes unconscious.
- Each new thrust should be a separate and distinct movement.[67,73,74,78]

Heimlich Maneuver With Victim Lying Down

- Place the victim in the supine position, face up (Fig 17).
- Kneel astride the victim's thighs and place the heel of one hand against the victim's abdomen, in the midline slightly above the navel and well below the tip of the xiphoid.
- Place the second hand directly on top of the first.
- Press into the abdomen with a quick upward thrust.

If you are in the correct position, you will have a natural midabdominal position and are thus unlikely to direct the thrust to the right or left. A rescuer too short to reach around the waist of an unconscious victim can use this technique. The rescuer can use his or her body weight to perform the maneuver.

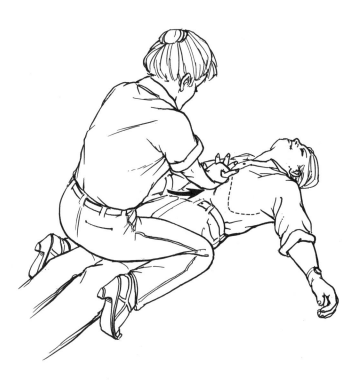

Fig 17. Heimlich maneuver administered to unconscious victim of foreign-body airway obstruction who is lying down.

The Self-administered Heimlich Maneuver

To treat one's own complete foreign-body airway obstruction:

- Make a fist with one hand.
- Place the thumb side on the abdomen above the navel and below the xiphoid process.
- Grasp the fist with the other hand.
- Press inward and upward toward the diaphragm with a quick motion.

If this is unsuccessful, press the upper abdomen quickly over any firm surface, such as the back of a chair, side of a table, or porch railing. Several thrusts may be needed to clear the airway.

Chest Thrusts With Victim Standing or Sitting

This technique is to be used only in the late stages of pregnancy or in the markedly obese victim.

- Stand behind the victim, with your arms directly under the victim's armpits, and encircle the victim's chest.
- Place the thumb side of your fist on the middle of

the victim's breastbone, taking care to avoid the xiphoid process and the margins of the rib cage.
- Grab your fist with the other hand and perform backward thrusts until the foreign body is expelled or the victim becomes unconscious.

Chest Thrusts With Victim Lying Down

This maneuver must be used only in the late stages of pregnancy and when the Heimlich maneuver cannot be applied effectively to the unconscious, markedly obese victim (Fig 18).

- Place the victim on his or her back and kneel close to the victim's side.
- The hand position for the application of chest thrusts is the same as that for chest compressions. In the adult, for example, the heel of the hand is on the lower half of the sternum.
- Deliver each thrust firmly and distinctly, with the intent of relieving the obstruction.

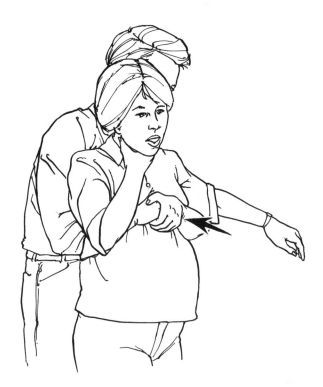

Fig 18. Chest thrust administered to a conscious victim (standing) of foreign body airway obstruction.

Finger Sweep

This maneuver should be used only in the unconscious victim, never in a seizure victim.

- With the victim's face up, open the victim's mouth by grasping both the tongue and lower jaw between the thumb and fingers and lifting the mandible (tongue-jaw lift). This action draws the tongue away from the back of the throat and away from a foreign body that may be lodged there. This alone may partially relieve the obstruction.
- Insert the index finger of the other hand down along the inside of the cheek and deeply into the throat to the base of the tongue.
- Use a hooking action to dislodge the foreign body and maneuver it into the mouth so that it can be removed (Fig 19).

It is sometimes necessary to use the index finger to push the foreign body against the opposite side of the throat to dislodge and remove it. Be careful not to force the object deeper into the airway. If the foreign body comes within reach, grasp and remove it.

Recommended Sequence for Victim Who Is or Becomes Unconscious

- Open the mouth of the unconscious victim. If you witness a victim losing consciousness and suspect that a foreign body is present, perform the finger sweep.

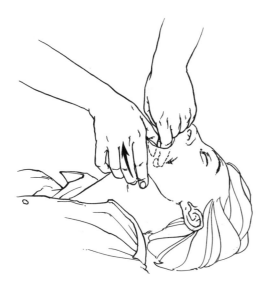

Fig 19. Finger sweep maneuver administered to an unconscious victim of foreign body airway obstruction.

- If the victim is found unconscious or no foreign body is suspected during witnessed unconsciousness, attempt rescue breathing.
- If unable to ventilate even after attempts to reposition the head, perform the Heimlich maneuver (up to five times).
- Open the mouth and perform a finger sweep.
- Attempt to ventilate.
- If unable to ventilate, reposition the head and try again to ventilate.
- Repeat the sequence of Heimlich maneuver, finger sweep, and attempt to ventilate.
- Persist in these efforts as long as necessary.
- If the victim resumes effective breathing, place him or her in the recovery position and monitor closely.
- Get appropriate medical attention.

General Recommendations

- The Heimlich maneuver is the recommended technique for relief of foreign-body airway obstruction in the adult. It may need to be repeated multiple times (for ease of teaching, *multiple* may be interpreted as up to five attempts). The use of only this method, which is at least as effective and as safe as any other single method, will simplify training programs and should result in better skills retention.
- It has previously been recommended that the chest thrust be used in the markedly obese person and in the late stages of pregnancy when there is no room between the enlarging uterus and the rib cage in which to perform abdominal thrusts.[74,79] Further investigation is necessary, and until such time, the chest thrust should remain as an alternative for the victim of foreign-body airway obstruction who is in advanced pregnancy or is markedly obese.
- As a single method, back blows may not be as effective as the Heimlich maneuver in adults.[69] For this reason and to simplify training, the Heimlich maneuver is the only method recommended at this time. More research and investigation are necessary.
- Under no circumstances should students practice the Heimlich maneuver on each other during CPR training.
- The use of devices to relieve foreign-body airway obstruction is restricted to persons properly trained in their application. The use of such devices by untrained or inexperienced persons is

unacceptable. Two types of conventional forceps are acceptable at present for foreign-body removal, the Kelly clamp and the Magill forceps. Both should be used only with direct visualization of the foreign body. Either a laryngoscope or tongue blade and flashlight can be used to permit direct visualization.

CPR: The Human Dimension

Since 1973, over 40 million people have learned CPR. Although considered by some to be the most successful public health initiative in recent times, the survival rate to hospital discharge averages 15%. This means that more than four out of five times, the efforts of rescuers who were taught to save lives are unsuccessful.

Serious long-lasting physical and emotional symptoms may occur in rescuers whose CPR efforts are unsuccessful. Rescuers may undergo grief reactions in much the same way as the family of the person who dies, displaying physical symptoms such as fatigue, difficulty sleeping, tight chest or tight throat, breathlessness, muscle weakness, headache, abdominal pain, and back pain. They may display emotional symptoms such as anxiety and depression.

Usually the physician is responsible for telling families that their loved ones have died, but rescuers should also know how to break bad news (Table 2).

Performance of CPR is stressful. The stress often leaves the rescuer feeling fatigued and uncertain, which may result in chronic anxiety, depression, and burnout. Burnout usually occurs when professional rescuers are subjected to repeated stress from unsuccessful CPR and have no opportunity to discuss their feelings. If CPR is part of a rescuer's job, it may lead to job dissatisfaction and the rescuer's choosing another career.

To decrease the chance of burnout and to allow rescuers to work through their feelings and their grief, a "critical incident debriefing" is recommended. Debriefings should be held after any unsuccessful CPR attempt. In these sessions rescuers discuss their thoughts, feelings, and performance. With the support of their coworkers they work through and express anxiety, guilt, anger, and other emotions they may have about the CPR attempt. Ideally all members of the resuscitation team should be present at the debriefing. A detailed analysis of what was done and why should occur, with a discussion of things that went right and things that went wrong. Everyone should be encouraged to ask questions about the CPR attempt and to discuss how things should or could have been done differently. The critical incident debriefing is also a time for learning something that may be useful next time.

All rescuers experience some anxiety. In most cases this is normal. The learning that occurs in stressful situations is in part through the anxiety experienced. Anxiety stimulates insight, and with feedback, education, clarification, and experience, leads to change and improvement.

The "human dimension" of CPR is often not discussed. Because of its importance it should be incorporated into CPR training and practice.

BLS Research Initiatives

The ongoing success and improvement of BLS programs require sound scientific research. Because of the lack of scientific data in some areas, many of the current guidelines are based on a consensus derived from limited published data, some clinical experience, and clinical judgment. Research in BLS is a fertile

---

Table 2. For the BLS Rescuer: Breaking Bad News to Families

You should know
- What happens to the body — who officially pronounces death, who signs the death certificate, and who calls the funeral home.
- How to contact local social workers or the clergy.

Before meeting family members or friends
- Make sure you know what happened during the resuscitation attempt and the sequence of events.

When meeting the family
- Take them to a quiet area, a separate room or a private office.
- Introduce yourself and explain your role in the resuscitative efforts.
- Sit down, rather than stand, if possible.
- Speak to the closest relative, describing what happened in as much detail as possible.
- Use specific words such as "death," "dying" or "dead." Avoid phrases such as "he's passed on," "she's no longer with us," or "he's left us."
- Maintain direct eye contact; state how you feel. It is acceptable to touch and to convey your sympathy.
- Encourage family members to ask questions. Give them time for sharing. Let them review the events several times to make sure they understand.
- The family may ask to see the body. Let them know if equipment is still connected or if there are signs of trauma.
- Offer to arrange follow-up or the aid of a social worker or clergyperson if one is not already present.
- Make sure the family knows what will happen next. If you are unsure, tell them you will find out. Write down important telephone numbers for further contact.

area for education, public health, and clinical and basic science investigators. During the 1992 National Conference on CPR and ECC, a number of potential areas of investigation were identified.

Barriers to CPR learning, various educational approaches to training, alternative BLS teaching aids, definition of populations being trained in CPR, training of the physically challenged, and the relation of the quality of CPR performance to patient outcome are challenges to education researchers.

EMS and public health investigators can improve BLS knowledge through studies of public awareness and action in obtaining early access to emergency medical systems. To facilitate this public awareness, it is important to learn how CPR is perceived and accepted by various socioeconomic and cultural groups.

It is important to emphasize the need for controlled scientific studies that evaluate all the present recommendations for ventilation and circulation. The impact and effectiveness of devices presently available for ventilation should be defined. Only through such studies can educated decisions be made for improvement of CPR.

Although knowledge has grown considerably in the last 25 years, BLS is a fundamental area of medical science with many more questions that remain to be investigated. Future changes and advances in CPR based on sound scientific investigation will likely improve the quality, delivery, and outcome of BLS.

References

1. *A Manual for Instructors in Basic Cardiac Life Support.* Dallas, Tex: American Heart Association; 1977.
2. Eisenberg MS, Bergner L, Hallstrom A. Cardiac resuscitation in the community: importance of rapid provision and implications for program planning. *JAMA.* 1979;241:1905-1907.
3. Cobb LA, Werner JA, Trobaugh GB. Sudden cardiac death: parts 1 and 2. *Mod Concepts Cardiovasc Dis.* 1980;49:31-36, 37-42.
4. Eisenberg MS, Copass MK, Hallstrom AP, et al. Treatment of out-of-hospital cardiac arrests with rapid defibrillation by emergency medical technicians. *N Engl J Med.* 1980;302: 1379-1383.
5. Myerburg RJ, Kessler KM, Zaman L, Conde CA, Castellanos A. Survivors of prehospital cardiac arrest. *JAMA.* 1982;247: 1485-1490.
6. Abramson NS, Safar P, Detre K, Kelsey S, Reinmuth O, Snyder J. An international collaborative clinical study mechanism for resuscitation research. *Resuscitation.* 1982;10:141-147.
7. Longstreth WT Jr, Diehr P, Inui TS. Prediction of awakening after out-of-hospital cardiac arrest. *N Engl J Med.* 1983;308: 1378-1382.
8. AHA Committee Report. Risk factors and coronary disease: a statement for physicians. *Circulation.* 1980;62:449A-455A.
9. Standards and guidelines for cardiopulmonary resuscitation (CPR) and emergency cardiac care (ECC). *JAMA.* 1986;255: 2905-2984.
10. Bayes de Luna A, Coumel P, Leclercq JF. Ambulatory sudden cardiac death: mechanisms of production of fatal arrhythmia on the basis of data from 157 cases. *Am Heart J.* 1989;117:151-159.
11. Eisenberg MS. Who shall live? Who shall die? In: Eisenberg MS, Bergner L, Hallstrom AP, eds. *Sudden Cardiac Death in the Community.* New York, NY: Praeger; 1984:44-58.
12. Weaver WD, Hill D, Fahrenbruch CE, et al. Use of the automatic external defibrillator in the management of out-of-hospital cardiac arrest. *N Engl J Med.* 1988;319:661-666.
13. Pepe P. Advanced cardiac life support: state of the art. In: Vincent JL, ed. *Emergency and Intensive Care.* New York, NY: Springer-Verlag NY Inc; 1990:565-585.
14. Eisenberg MS, Copass MK, Hallstrom AP, et al. Treatment of out-of-hospital cardiac arrests with rapid defibrillation by emergency medical technicians. *N Engl J Med.* 1980;302: 1379-1383.
15. Stults KR, Brown DD, Schug VL, Bean JA. Prehospital defibrillation performed by emergency medical technicians in rural communities. *N Engl J Med.* 1984;310:219-223.
16. Vukov LF, White RD, Bachman JW, O'Brien PC. New perspectives on rural EMT defibrillation. *Ann Emerg Med.* 1988;17:318-321.
17. Bachman JW, McDonald GS, O'Brien PC. A study of out-of-hospital cardiac arrests in northeastern Minnesota. *JAMA.* 1986;256:477-483.
18. Olson DW, LaRochelle J, Fark D, et al. EMT-defibrillation: the Wisconsin experience. *Ann Emerg Med.* 1989;18:806-811.
19. Cummins RO, Eisenberg MS, Hallstrom AP, Litwin PE. Survival of out-of-hospital cardiac arrest with early initiation of cardiopulmonary resuscitation. *Am J Emerg Med.* 1985;3: 114-119.
20. Walters G, Glucksman E. Planning a pre-hospital cardiac resuscitation programme: an analysis of community and system factors in London. *J R Coll Physicians Lond.* 1989;23:107-110.
21. Stults KR. Phone first. *J Emerg Med Serv.* 1987;12:28.
22. Improving survival from sudden cardiac arrest: the 'chain of survival' concept. A statement for health professionals from the Advanced Cardiac Life Support Subcommittee and the Emergency Cardiac Care Committee, American Heart Association: Cummins RO, Ornato JP, Thies WH, Pepe PE. *Circulation.* 1991;83:1832-1847. Special report.
23. National Association of EMS Physicians. Emergency medical dispatching. *Prehosp Disaster Med.* 1989;4:163-166. Position paper.
24. Clawson JJ. Dispatch priority training: strengthening the weak link. *J Emerg Med Serv.* 1981;6:32-36.
25. Clawson JJ. Telephone treatment protocols: reach out and help someone. *J Emerg Med Serv.* 1986;11:43-46.
26. Culley LL, Clark JJ, Eisenberg MS, Larsen MP. Dispatcher-assisted telephone CPR: common delays and time standards for delivery. *Ann Emerg Med.* 1991;20:362-366.
27. *Standard Practice for Emergency Medical Dispatch.* Philadelphia, Pa: American Society for Testing and Materials; 1990. Publication F1258-90.
28. Zaritsky A, Nadkarni V, Getson P, Kuehl K. CPR in children. *Ann Emerg Med.* 1987;16:1107-1111.

29. Safar P. The pathology of dying and reanimation. In: Schwartz GR, ed. *Principles and Practice of Emergency Medicine*. 2nd ed. Philadelphia, Pa: WB Saunders Co; 1986.

30. *Instructor's Manual for Basic Life Support*. Dallas, Tex: American Heart Association; 1985.

31. Safar P. Ventilatory efficacy of mouth-to-mouth artificial respiration: airway obstruction during manual and mouth-to-mouth artificial respiration. *JAMA*. 1958;167:335-341.

32. Safar P, Escarraga LA, Chang F. Upper airway obstruction in the unconscious patient. *J Appl Physiol*. 1959;14:760-764.

33. Morikawa S, Safar P, DeCarlo J. Influence of the head-jaw position upon upper airway patency. *Anesthesiology*. 1961;22:265-270.

34. Ruben HM, Elam JO, Ruben AM, Greene DG. Investigation of upper airway problems in resuscitation, I: studies of pharyngeal x-rays and performance by laymen. *Anesthesiology*. 1961;22:271-279.

35. Boidin MP. Airway patency in the unconscious patient. *Br J Anaesth*. 1985;57:306-310.

36. Guildner CW. Resuscitation–opening the airway: a comparative study of techniques for opening an airway obstructed by the tongue. *J Am Coll Emerg Phys*. 1976;5:588-590.

37. Safar P. *Cardiopulmonary Cerebral Resuscitation*. Philadelphia, Pa: WB Saunders Co; 1981.

38. Elam JO, Greene DG, Schneider MA, et al. Head-tilt method of oral resuscitation. *JAMA*. 1960;172:812-815.

39. Safar P, Lind B. Triple airway maneuver, artificial ventilation and oxygen inhalation by mouth-to-mask and bag-valve-mask techniques. In: *Proceedings of the National Conference on Standards for Cardiopulmonary Resuscitation (CPR) and Emergency Cardiac Care (ECC)*. Dallas, Tex: American Heart Association; 1975.

40. Greene DG, Elam JO, Dobkin AB, Studley CL. Cinefluorographic study of hyperextension of the neck and upper airway patency. *JAMA*. 1961;176:570-573.

41. Elam JO, Greene DG. Mission accomplished: successful mouth-to-mouth resuscitation. *Anesth Analg*. 1961;40:440-442,578-580,672-676.

42. Ruben H, Knudsen EJ, Carugati G. Gastric inflation in relation to airway pressure. *Acta Anaesthesiol Scand*. 1961;5:107-114.

43. Melker RJ. Asynchronous and other alternative methods of ventilation during CPR. *Ann Emerg Med*. 1984;13(pt 2):758-761.

44. Melker RJ. Recommendations for ventilation during cardiopulmonary resuscitation: time for change? *Crit Care Med*. 1985;13(pt 2):882-883.

45. Ruben H. The immediate treatment of respiratory failure. *Br J Anaesth*. 1964;36:542-549.

46. Safar P, Redding J. The 'tight jaw' in resuscitation. *Anesthesiology*. 1959;20:701-702.

47. International Association of Laryngectomees. *First Aid for (Neck Breathers) Laryngectomees*. New York, NY: American Cancer Society; 1971.

48. Sellick BA. Cricoid pressure to control regurgitation of stomach contents during induction of anesthesia. *Lancet*. 1961;2:404-406.

49. Petito SP, Russell WJ. The prevention of gastric inflation: a neglected benefit of cricoid pressure. *Anaesth Intensive Care*. 1988;16:139-143.

50. Salem MR, Wong AY, Mani M, Sellick BA. Efficacy of cricoid pressure in preventing gastric inflation during bag-mask ventilation in pediatric patients. *Anesthesiology*. 1974;40:96-98.

51. Kouwenhoven WB, Jude JR, Knickerbocker GG. Closed-chest cardiac massage. *JAMA*. 1960;173:1064-1067.

52. Maier GW, Tyson GS Jr, Olsen CO, et al. The physiology of external cardiac massage: high-impulse cardiopulmonary resuscitation. *Circulation*. 1984;70:86-101.

53. Rudikoff MT, Maughan WL, Effron M, Freund P, Weisfeldt ML. Mechanisms of blood flow during cardiopulmonary resuscitation. *Circulation*. 1980;61:345-352.

54. Safar P, Brown TC, Holtey WJ, Wilder RJ. Ventilation and circulation with closed-chest cardiac massage in man. *JAMA*. 1961;176:574-576.

55. Babbs CF. New versus old theories of blood flow during CPR. *Crit Care Med*. 1980;8:191-195.

56. Feneley MP, Maier GW, Gaynor JW, et al. Sequence of mitral valve motion and transmitral blood flow during manual cardiopulmonary resuscitation in dogs. *Circulation*. 1987;76:363-375.

57. Deshmukh HG, Weil MH, Gudipati CV, Trevino RP, Bisera J, Rackow EC. Mechanism of blood flow generated by precordial compression during CPR, I: studies on closed chest precordial compression. *Chest*. 1989;95:1092-1099.

58. Werner JA, Greene HL, Janko CL, Cobb LA. Visualization of cardiac valve motion in man during external chest compression using two-dimensional echocardiography: implications regarding the mechanism of blood flow. *Circulation*. 1981;63:1417-1421.

59. Niemann JT, Rosborough JP, Hausknecht M, Garner D, Criley JM. Pressure-synchronized cineangiography during experimental cardiopulmonary resuscitation. *Circulation*. 1981;64:985-991.

60. Weisfeldt ML, Halperin HR. Cardiopulmonary resuscitation: beyond cardiac massage. *Circulation*. 1986;74:443-448.

61. Criley JM, Blaufuss AH, Kissel GL. Cough-induced cardiac compression: self-administered form of cardiopulmonary resuscitation. *JAMA*. 1976;236:1246-1250.

62. Paradis NA, Martin GB, Goetting MG, et al. Simultaneous aortic, jugular bulb, and right atrial pressures during cardiopulmonary resuscitation in humans: insights into mechanisms. *Circulation*. 1989;80:361-368.

63. Halperin HR, Weiss JL, Guerci AD, et al. Cyclic elevation of intrathoracic pressure can close the mitral valve during cardiac arrest in dogs. *Circulation*. 1988;78:754-760.

64. Porter TR, Ornato JP, Guard CS, Roy VG, Burns CA, Nixon JV. Transesophageal echocardiography to assess mitral valve function and flow during cardiopulmonary resuscitation. *Am J Cardiol*. 1992;70:1056-1060.

65. Neimann JT, Rosborough J, Hausknecht M, Brown D, Criley JM. Cough-CPR: documentation of systemic perfusion in man and in an experimental model: a 'window' to the mechanism of blood flow in external CPR. *Crit Care Med*. 1980;8:141-146.

66. National Safety Council. *Accident Facts 1989*. Chicago, Ill: National Safety Council; 1989.

67. Haugen RK. The café coronary: sudden death in restaurants. *JAMA*. 1963;186:142-143.

68. Heimlich HJ. A life-saving maneuver to prevent food-choking. *JAMA*. 1975;234:398-401.

69. Day RL, Crelin ES, DuBois AB. Choking: the Heimlich abdominal thrust vs back blows: an approach to measurement of inertial and aerodynamic forces. *Pediatrics*. 1982;70:113-119.

70. Day RL, DuBois AB. Treatment of choking. *Pediatrics.* 1983;71:300-301.

71. Day RL. Differing opinions on the emergency treatment of choking. *Pediatrics.* 1983;71:976-978.

72. Patrick EA. *Decision Analysis in Medicine: Methods and Applications.* Boca Raton, Fla: CRC Press Inc; 1979;90-93.

73. Heimlich HJ, Hoffmann KA, Canestri FR. Food-choking and drowning deaths prevented by external subdiaphragmatic compression: physiological basis. *Ann Thorac Surg.* 1975;20:188-195.

74. Heimlich HJ, Uhley MH, Netter FH. The Heimlich maneuver. *Clin Symp.* 1979;31:1-32.

75. Patrick EA. Choking: a questionnaire to find the most effective treatment. *Emergency.* 1980;12:59-64.

76. Visintine RE, Baick CH. Ruptured stomach after Heimlich maneuver. *JAMA.* 1975;234:415.

77. Palmer ED. The Heimlich maneuver misused. *Curr Prescribing.* 1979;5:45-49.

78. Heimlich HJ. Pop goes the cafe coronary. *Emerg Med.* 1974;6:154-155.

79. Standards and guidelines for cardiopulmonary resuscitation (CPR) and emergency cardiac care (ECC). *JAMA.* 1980; 244:453-509.

Special Resuscitation Situations

Chapter 5

Cardiopulmonary arrest is not always cardiac in origin. A number of situations can lead to cardiopulmonary arrest, and rescuers may need to change their approach to resuscitation in these special circumstances. Some of the more common special resuscitation situations are stroke, seizures, hypothermia, near-drowning, injury, electric shock, lightning strike, and pregnancy. This section discusses the differences in emphasis, technique, and triage in these situations.

Stroke

Stroke is the third leading cause of death in the United States, ranking behind heart attack and all forms of cancer. Some 2 980 000 Americans now alive have been stroke victims. In 1991 approximately 500 000 new and recurrent cases of stroke occurred, resulting in 144 070 deaths from complications of stroke (Fig 1).

Stroke is an illness of sudden onset caused by occlusion or rupture of a blood vessel that supplies the brain. Approximately 75% of strokes are ischemic: an artery is blocked by a blood clot that either developed within the vessel (thrombosis) or arose from another source, usually the heart, and migrated to the brain (embolism). Hemorrhagic stroke is the result of a ruptured brain blood vessel. The bleeding can occur adjacent to the brain (subarachnoid hemorrhage) or into the substance of the brain (intracerebral hemorrhage).

In many cases stroke can be prevented, but only if warning signs are heeded. An important forecaster of ischemic stroke is a brief, reversible episode of focal neurological dysfunction called a *transient ischemic attack* (TIA). Effective medical and surgical therapies may prevent stroke in these cases, but the key to success is prompt recognition and rapid initiation of therapy.[2-5]

Unfortunately some strokes occur without warning and may rapidly result in brain damage. Acute stroke may be treatable; several medical and surgical treatments may reduce the consequences of stroke.[6-8] Early intervention can also prevent neurological or general medical complications of stroke. *Therefore, evaluation and management must be undertaken quickly to achieve the best possible result in stroke patients.*

Risk Factors for Stroke

The best way to prevent a stroke is to reduce the risk factors for stroke. Some factors that increase the risk of stroke are genetically determined, while others cannot be changed. Some risk factors can be modified under the direction of a physician.

Risk Factors That Can Be Changed

Modifiable risk factors include high blood pressure, heart disease, cigarette smoking, high red blood cell count, and transient ischemic attacks.

High Blood Pressure. Hypertension is the most important risk factor for stroke. It afflicts almost one in three American adults. For this reason everyone should have his or her blood pressure checked regularly. Controlling high blood pressure reduces the risk of stroke significantly. Often blood pressure can be controlled simply by eating a healthier diet and maintaining proper weight. Drugs to control blood pressure are also available. It is thought that the death rate from stroke has declined over the past decade because of better control of high blood pressure.

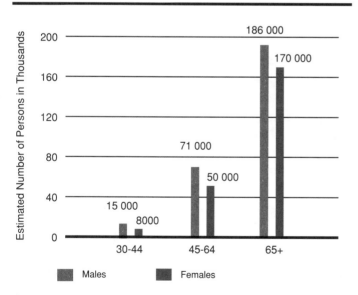

Source: Framingham Heart Study, 24-year follow-up.

Fig 1. Estimated annual number of Americans, by age and gender, experiencing stroke — age 30 and older.[1]

Heart Disease. A diseased heart increases the risk of stroke. Independent of blood pressure, people with heart problems have more than twice the risk of stroke than people with normally functioning hearts. The three major controllable risk factors for heart attacks are cigarette smoking, elevated blood cholesterol, and high blood pressure. Controlling these factors reduces the risk of heart disease and thus the risk of stroke.

Cigarette Smoking. Cigarette smoking is an important risk factor for stroke. Smoking damages the cardiovascular system. Nicotine increases blood pressure. Carbon monoxide reduces the amount of oxygen the blood can supply to the body. Cigarette smoking also causes blood platelets to cluster, shortens platelet survival, decreases clotting time, and increases blood thickness.

High Red Blood Cell Count. A marked or even moderate increase in the red blood cell count is a risk factor for stroke because increased red blood cells thicken the blood and make clots more likely. This problem is treatable by removing blood or administering blood thinners.

Transient Ischemic Attacks (TIAs). Only about 10% of strokes are preceded by TIAs. Nevertheless, TIAs are extremely important; they are strong predictors of stroke. TIAs are usually treated with drugs that inhibit formation of clots.

Risk Factors That Cannot Be Changed

Risk factors for stroke that cannot be changed are age, gender, race, diabetes mellitus, prior stroke, heredity, and asymptomatic carotid bruit.

Age. Incidence of stroke is strongly related to age. In fact, for people aged 55 years and older, the incidence of stroke more than doubles in each successive decade. A common misconception is that only elderly people suffer strokes. About 28% of stroke victims in a given year are less than 65 years old. Older people do have a much greater risk of stroke than younger people. The risk of stroke in people aged 65 to 74 is about 1% a year. If they have had a TIA, however, it increases to 5% to 8% a year.

Gender. The incidence of stroke is about 19% higher for men than for women. For people under age 65, the difference is greater still.

Race. African-Americans have a much greater risk of death and disability from stroke than Caucasians. This may be because African-Americans have a greater incidence of high blood pressure.

Diabetes Mellitus. Although diabetes is treatable, persons who have it are much more likely to suffer a stroke. This association is greater in women than

men. Many times diabetics also have hypertension, increasing their risk of stroke even more.

Prior Stroke. The risk of stroke for someone who has already had one is many times that of someone who has not.

Heredity. Risk of stroke is greater for people who have a family history of stroke.

Asymptomatic Carotid Bruit. A bruit is an abnormal sound heard when a stethoscope is placed over an artery (in this case, the carotid artery, which is in the neck). A bruit often indicates partial obstruction (atherosclerosis) of an artery and may be associated with an increased risk of stroke.

Other Risk Factors

Besides the risk factors listed, other (controllable) factors indirectly increase stroke risk. These include elevated blood cholesterol and lipids, excessive alcohol intake, physical inactivity, and obesity. These are secondary risk factors because they affect the risk of stroke indirectly by increasing the risk of heart disease, which is a primary risk factor for stroke.

Finally, it is worth noting that some rather low-level risk factors become extremely significant when combined with certain other risk factors. Taking oral contraceptives and smoking cigarettes, for example, increases the risk of stroke considerably in young women. More to the point, a large population of stroke victims have a set of five risk factors. These are

- High blood pressure
- Elevated blood cholesterol levels
- High blood sugar (abnormal glucose tolerance)
- Cigarette smoking
- Left ventricular hypertrophy (enlarged heart)

People who have all these risk factors should have close medical supervision.

Clinical Presentation

Stroke should be suspected in any patient with sudden loss of neurological function or alteration in consciousness. The symptoms of stroke, outlined in Table 1, can occasionally occur alone or in any combination. The findings can be most severe at the beginning, wax and wane, or worsen progressively. The clinical presentations of ischemic and hemorrhagic stroke overlap. Thus, emergency personnel should not depend solely on symptoms for diagnosis. In general, headaches (often described by victims as "the worst headache of my life"), disturbances in consciousness,

Table 1. Clinical Presentation of Acute Stroke

Alteration in consciousness (coma, stupor, confusion, seizures, delirium)

Intense or unusually severe headache of sudden onset or any headache associated with decreased level of consciousness or neurological deficit; unusual and severe neck or facial pain

Aphasia (incoherent speech or difficulty understanding speech)

Facial weakness or asymmetry (paralysis of the facial muscles, usually noted when the patient speaks or smiles); may be on the same side or opposite side from limb paralysis

Incoordination, weakness, paralysis, or sensory loss of one or more limbs; usually involves one half of the body and in particular the hand

Ataxia (poor balance, clumsiness, or difficulty walking)

Visual loss (monocular or binocular); may be a partial loss of visual field

Dysarthria (slurred or indistinct speech)

Intense vertigo, double vision, unilateral hearing loss, nausea, vomiting, photophobia, or phonophobia

---

nausea, and vomiting are more prominent with intracranial hemorrhages. Loss of consciousness may be transient with resolution by the time the patient receives medical attention. Patients with subarachnoid hemorrhage may have an intense headache without focal neurological signs.

Initial Examination of the Stroke Patient

The evaluation (examination and baseline diagnostic studies) should be done as quickly as possible — 1 hour is the goal.

Airway

Airway obstruction may be a major problem in acute stroke if the patient is comatose. Because poor ventilation and inadequate oxygenation can make a stroke worse, inadequate ventilation or aspiration is a serious concern. An adequate airway must be established and maintained and endotracheal intubation performed if necessary.

Vital Signs

Vital signs (pulse, respirations, and blood pressure) should be checked frequently to detect abnormalities and changes (Table 2). Disturbances of vital signs are common after stroke. Abnormal respirations often occur in comatose patients and may indicate serious brain dysfunction.[9] Hypertension (high blood pressure) is often found after stroke and may represent previously unrecognized underlying hypertension, a stress reaction to the condition, or a normal response to

decreased brain blood flow. In such victims blood pressure often returns to normal without treatment. Hypotension (a fall in blood pressure) is rarely due to stroke, and other causes should be considered. Continuous noninvasive blood pressure monitoring is recommended for the first few hours after hemorrhagic stroke. Cardiac arrhythmias can occur in stroke victims and may be the consequence of brain injury or may point to an underlying cardiac cause of embolism to the brain. Life-threatening cardiac arrhythmias are an important early complication of stroke, particularly of intracranial hemorrhages.[10] Continuous monitoring of cardiac rhythm should be part of the early assessment of a stroke patient.

General Medical Assessment

The patient should be examined for any evidence of injury to the head or neck because trauma is important in the differential (alternative) diagnoses of stroke.

Neurological Assessment

Clinical assessments of the neurological status of the patient (Table 2) should be done frequently to detect any change. The examination need not be exhaustive. The most important feature is the patient's level of consciousness. Depressed consciousness represents a major brain injury and identifies stroke patients most at risk of dying in the next few hours. The Glasgow Coma Scale (Table 3) is particularly important for appraising the severity of neurological deficits in patients with altered consciousness and is useful in rating the severity of stroke.[11]

Table 2. Assessment of the Patient With Acute Stroke

Ensure adequate airway

Measure vital signs frequently

Conduct general medical assessment

    Trauma of head or neck

    Cardiovascular abnormalities

    Ocular signs

    Other signs

Conduct neurological examination

    Level of consciousness

    Glasgow Coma Scale (score 3-15)[11]

    Pupils

    Individual limb movements

    Meningeal signs

Table 3. Glasgow Coma Scale

Eye opening	
Spontaneous	4
To speech	3
To pain	2
None	1
Best motor response	
Obeys	6
Localizes	5
Withdraws	4
Abnormal flexion	3
Abnormal extension	2
None	1
Best verbal response	
Oriented conversation	5
Confused conversation	4
Inappropriate words	3
Incomprehensible sounds	2
None	1

Diagnosis of Stroke

The differential diagnosis of stroke is not extensive; few neurological illnesses have a similar sudden course (Fig 2). The number of alternative diagnoses is larger when the patient is comatose or when no history of the current illness is available. Hypoglycemia (low blood sugar) can cause focal neurological deficits without a major alteration in consciousness and is an important consideration in a diabetic patient with stroke. Seizures can be unwitnessed, and the patient may be found with only focal neurological signs after the seizure (the postictal period) that can last several hours. Patients with stroke may fall, which may cause a head injury, or patients who fall and sustain head injuries may have had a stroke.

Ambulance or emergency department personnel should evaluate airway and breathing. It is also important to test blood glucose, particularly in a diabetic patient, although the test should not delay other treatment. Glucose may be administered if hypoglycemia is strongly suspected.

General Emergency Therapy

In victims of stroke, general emergency therapy will usually focus on maintaining airway patency. Because of loss of muscle tone and paralysis, upper airway occlusion can occur and present as "noisy" obstructed breathing, or in more extreme cases the victim will develop a bluish discoloration around the lips and in

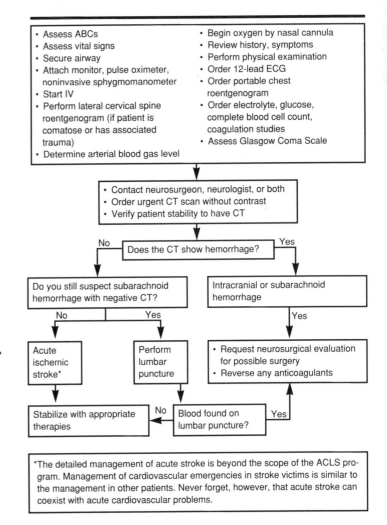

*The detailed management of acute stroke is beyond the scope of the ACLS program. Management of cardiovascular emergencies in stroke victims is similar to the management in other patients. Never forget, however, that acute stroke can coexist with acute cardiovascular problems.

Fig 2. Algorithm for initial evaluation of suspected stroke.

the nail beds (cyanosis). In such situations, the airway should be opened (head tilt–chin lift), and if there is no breathing, rescue breathing should be started. Seizures are a potential complication of acute stroke, and in some instances they are recurrent. Recurrent seizures can worsen the consequences of stroke and should be stopped promptly. Protection of the airway, supplemental oxygen, and maintenance of normal body temperature are an essential part of supportive care.

For further, more detailed discussion of stroke management, refer to the *Textbook of Advanced Cardiac Life Support,* chapter 10.

Seizure

Although seizures can occur in stroke victims, there are many other causes of seizures. Seizures may or may not be convulsive. Nonconvulsive seizures include (1) staring attacks with loss of awareness for a few seconds, called *absence seizures* (older term:

petit mal), and (2) attacks of confusion and loss of awareness with semipurposeful behavior lasting a few minutes, called *complex partial seizures.* No first-aid procedures are required for these seizures, but close observation is recommended. Of the convulsive seizures, the generalized tonoclonic or grand mal is the most easily recognized since the person may suddenly fall to the floor and convulse.

Convulsions as a consequence of cardiac arrest can simulate grand mal seizures. Seizures are distinguished from convulsions associated with cardiac arrest by the presence of pulse and blood pressure and by the return of breathing at the termination of the episode. Treatment of a convulsive seizure requires protection of the head, observation during and after the seizure, and at the termination turning the person to the recovery position to allow pooled secretions to clear. *Objects should not be placed in the mouth, and movements should not be restrained.* Aspiration of food may occur as a complication of any seizure and may require treatment.

The most important action is to protect the victim:

- Cradle or place something soft under the victim's head (such as a towel or your hands) to prevent head injury.
- Remove all sharp or dangerous objects that are nearby.

Convulsive seizures run their course, and a bystander can do nothing to prevent or terminate an attack. After the seizure

- Assess airway and breathing
- Make sure the mouth is cleared of food and saliva
- If breathing is adequate, place the victim in the recovery position

Incontinence (loss of urinary or fecal control) is common during a seizure. If the rescuer remains calm, the person will be reassured when alertness is resumed. Do not put liquids into the victim's mouth or offer any food, drink, or medication until the victim is fully awake. If repeated attacks occur or if the seizure lasts longer than a few minutes, activate the EMS system to transport the victim to a medical facility.

Breathing almost always resumes spontaneously after a convulsive seizure. Otherwise, a complication of the seizure has occurred, such as the aspiration of food, an associated heart attack, or severe head or neck injury. In this case, CPR should be initiated. Rarely, sudden death may follow an epileptic seizure and is thought to be secondary to ventricular fibrillation (VF). The same resuscitative measures used for sudden death from coronary heart disease should be followed.

Hypothermia

Severe hypothermia (body temperature below 30°C [86°F]) is associated with marked depression of cerebral blood flow and oxygen requirement, reduced cardiac output, and decreased arterial pressure. Victims can appear to be clinically dead because of marked depression of brain function. Full resuscitation with intact neurological recovery may be possible, although unusual.[12] The victim's peripheral pulses and respiratory efforts may be difficult to detect, but lifesaving procedures should not be withheld based on clinical presentation. Victims should be transported as soon as possible to a center where monitored rewarming is possible.

If the victim is not breathing, rescue breathing should be initiated. In the pulseless patient CPR should be started immediately, although pulse and respirations may need to be checked for longer periods to detect minimal cardiopulmonary efforts. The traditional recommendation that pulse and respirations be checked for 1 to 2 minutes before beginning CPR[13,14] is excessive. A period of 30 to 45 seconds confirms pulselessness or bradycardia profound enough for CPR to be initiated. To prevent further core heat loss from the victim, remove wet garments from the victim, insulate or shield him or her from wind, heat, or cold, and if possible ventilate with warm, humidified oxygen.[12,15] For victims not in cardiac arrest, it is appropriate to apply external warming devices to truncal areas only (warm packs to neck, armpits, and groin). After stabilization, the patient should be carefully prepared for transport to a hospital. All other field interventions require ACLS capability.

Core temperature determinations in the field with either tympanic membrane sensors or rectal probes are recommended (for EMS systems so equipped) but should not delay transfer. The patient should be handled carefully during transportation to prevent VF and transported in the horizontal position to avoid aggravating hypotension.

If the hypothermic victim is in cardiac arrest, the usual treatment protocol should be followed. Automated external defibrillators should be available on virtually all BLS rescue units, and if VF is detected, emergency personnel should be allowed to deliver three shocks to determine fibrillation responsiveness. If VF persists after three shocks, efforts to defibrillate should cease and emergency personnel should immediately begin CPR, rewarming, and stabilization for transportation. If core temperature is below 30°C (86°F), successful conversion to normal sinus rhythm may not be possible until rewarming is accomplished.[16]

Some clinicians believe that patients who appear dead after prolonged exposure to cold temperatures should not be considered dead until they are near normal core temperature and are still unresponsive to CPR.[17] Successful resuscitation may be more difficult if drowning preceded hypothermia. If the arrest was unwitnessed, emergency personnel and hospital providers will not know if the arrest was due to hypothermia or if hypothermia was a sequel to a normothermic arrest. For example, a middle-aged man who has a normothermic cardiac arrest while shoveling snow may cool down after the arrest. When it is not clinically possible to know which event occurred first, rescuers should attempt to stabilize the patient with CPR, and if hypothermia is documented, should initiate basic maneuvers to limit heat loss and aid with rewarming. Physicians in the hospital should use their clinical judgment to decide when resuscitative efforts should cease in a hypothermic arrest victim.

Severe accidental hypothermia is a serious and preventable health problem. Hypothermia in inner-city areas has a high association with poverty and drug and alcohol use.[18,19] In some rural areas, over 90% of hypothermic deaths are associated with elevated blood alcohol levels.[20] Successful treatment of hypothermia requires optimal training of emergency personnel and appropriate resuscitation methods at each institution.

Near-Drowning

The most important consequence of prolonged underwater submersion without ventilation is hypoxemia. The duration of hypoxia is the critical factor in determining the victim's outcome. Therefore, restoration of ventilation and perfusion should be accomplished as rapidly as possible. This requires immediate initiation of BLS support and the prompt activation of the EMS system.

Rescue From the Water

When attempting to rescue a near-drowning victim, the rescuer should get to the victim as quickly as possible, preferably with some conveyance (boat, raft, surfboard, or flotation device). The rescuer must always be aware of personal safety in attempting a rescue and should exercise caution to minimize the danger.

Rescue Breathing

Initial treatment of the near-drowning victim consists of rescue breathing with the mouth-to-mouth technique. Rescue breathing should be started as soon as the victim's airway can be opened and protected and the rescuer's safety can be ensured. This is usually achieved when the victim is in shallow water or out of the water.

If neck injury is suspected, the victim's neck should be maintained in a neutral position (without flexion or extension), and the victim should be floated supine onto a horizontal back support before being removed from the water. If the victim must be turned, the head, neck, chest, and body should be aligned, supported, and turned as a unit to the horizontal, supine position. Rescue breathing should be provided with the head maintained in a neutral position; ie, jaw thrust without head tilt or chin lift without head tilt should be used.

Rescue breathing should be initiated immediately if the submersion victim is not breathing. Management of the airway and breathing of the submersion victim are similar to those of any victim in cardiopulmonary arrest. There is no need to clear the airway of aspirated water. At most, only a modest amount of water is aspirated by the majority of drowning victims.[21] Furthermore, some victims do not aspirate at all because of laryngospasm or breath-holding.[21,22] An attempt to remove water from the breathing passages by any means other than suction is usually unnecessary and apt to be dangerous because it is likely to eject gastric contents and cause aspiration.[22]

A Heimlich maneuver delays initiation of ventilation and breathing. Its value is not proven scientifically and is supported only by anecdotal evidence, and its risk-benefit ratio is untested. Therefore, a Heimlich maneuver should be used only if the rescuer suspects that foreign matter is obstructing the airway or if the victim does not respond appropriately to mouth-to-mouth ventilation. Then, if necessary, CPR should be resumed after the Heimlich maneuver has been performed.[23-25] The Heimlich maneuver is performed on the near-drowning victim as described in the treatment of foreign-body airway obstruction (unconscious supine) except that the victim's head should be turned sideways unless cervical trauma is suspected.

Chest Compressions

Chest compressions should not be attempted in the water. It is usually not possible to keep the victim's body horizontal and the head above water in position for CPR.

After removal from the water, the victim must be immediately assessed for adequacy of circulation. The pulse may be difficult to appreciate in a near-drowning victim because of impaired heart function. If a pulse cannot be felt, chest compressions should be started at once.

General Considerations

Every submersion victim, even one who requires only minimal resuscitation and regains consciousness at the scene, should be transferred to a medical facility for follow-up care. Pulmonary injury may develop as late as several hours after submersion. In such victims hypothermia is common and should be addressed using techniques discussed earlier in this chapter.

Although survival is unlikely in victims who have undergone prolonged submersion and require prolonged resuscitation,[26] successful resuscitation with full neurological recovery has infrequently occurred in near-drowning victims with prolonged submersion in extremely cold water.[17,27,28] There is no established time limit for when resuscitative efforts should be withheld. Since it is often difficult for rescuers to obtain an accurate time of submersion, attempts at resuscitation should be initiated by rescuers at the scene unless there is obvious physical evidence of death (such as putrefaction). The victim should be transported with continued CPR to an advanced life support facility where a physician can decide whether to continue resuscitation. Aggressive attempts at resuscitation in the hospital should be continued for the victim of cold water submersion.

Cardiac Arrest Associated With Trauma

General Considerations

The initial treatment of the patient who develops cardiac arrest after an injury does not differ from care of the patient with a primary cardiac or respiratory arrest. Cardiopulmonary arrest associated with trauma has several possible causes, and the management plan may vary.

These causes include

- Severe brain or spinal cord injury with secondary cardiovascular collapse
- Hypoxia secondary to respiratory arrest resulting from brain stem or spinal cord injury, airway obstruction, collapse of the lungs (pneumothorax), or severe airway laceration or crush
- Direct and severe injury to vital structures that sustain cardiovascular function, such as the heart, aorta, or upper and lower airways
- Underlying medical problems that led to the injury, such as sudden VF in the driver of a motor vehicle or the victim of an electric shock
- Severely diminished cardiac output from tension pneumothorax or pericardial tamponade (bleeding into the fibrous sac that surrounds the heart)
- Hemorrhage leading to severe blood loss and severely diminished oxygen delivery
- Injuries in a cold environment (eg, fractured leg) complicated by secondary severe hypothermia

If cardiac arrest occurs in victims of blunt or penetrating trauma, the prognosis is poor. However, there is potential for reversibility and long-term survival in certain cases of respiratory arrest through aggressive early airway management and ventilatory support. Such interventions, however, must occur early in the prehospital setting. Underlying VF may be treatable with early defibrillation.

Studies show that patients who survive prehospital cardiopulmonary arrest associated with trauma generally (1) are young with penetrating injuries, (2) have received early (prehospital) endotracheal intubation, and (3) undergo prompt transport by highly skilled paramedics to a definitive care facility.[29,30]

Specific Prehospital Approaches to Cardiac Arrest Associated With Injuries

Rapid extrication and rapid transport to a trauma center are essential for the successful resuscitation of the entrapped victim. Airway assessment and ventilation should be accomplished as soon as possible. During airway procedures, an assistant should immobilize the neck.[31] Lateral neck supports, strapping, and use of backboards are also recommended to minimize exacerbation of an occult neck injury.[32]

Chest compressions are of unknown value in the victims of trauma-associated cardiac arrest. Compressions were used in two studies that demonstrated favorable outcomes following prehospital arrest.[29,30] Intuitively, chest compressions in this circumstance should have limited effect given the possible causes of the cardiac arrest (pericardial tamponade or exsanguinating hemorrhage). Chest compressions can be initiated for pulseless trauma patients, but preferably after defibrillation and airway control are provided.[32] When an automated defibrillator is available, it can be safely used.

Electric Shock and Lightning Strike

Electric Shock

Electric shock is associated with a fatality rate of 0.5 per 100 000 population per year in the United States. It accounts for approximately 500 to 1000 deaths annually in the United States and causes an additional 5000 patients to require emergency treatment.[33-35] Victims of electric shock experience a wide spectrum of injury, ranging from a transient unpleasant sensation from low-intensity current to instantaneous cardiac arrest from accidental electrocution.

Electric shock injuries result from the direct effects of current and the conversion of electric energy into heat energy as current passes through body tissues. Factors that determine the nature and severity of electric trauma include the magnitude of energy delivered, resistance to current flow, type of current, duration of contact with the current source, and current pathway. High-tension current generally causes the most serious injuries, although fatal electrocutions may occur with low-voltage household current (110 V).[36] Bone and skin are most resistant to the passage of electric current; muscle, blood vessels, and nerves conduct with least resistance.[34,35] Skin resistance, the most important factor impeding current flow, can be reduced substantially by moisture, thereby converting what ordinarily might be a minor low-voltage injury into a life-threatening shock.[37] Alternating current at 60 cycles per second (the frequency used in most household and commercial sources of electricity) is substantially more dangerous than direct current of the same magnitude. Contact with alternating current may cause tetanic skeletal muscle contractions, which prevent the victim from releasing the source of the electricity and lead to increased delivery of current.

Transthoracic current flow (eg, a hand-to-hand pathway) is more likely to be fatal than a vertical (hand-to-foot) or straddle (foot-to-foot) current path.[38] However, the vertical pathway often causes increased cardiac damage, possibly because of longer electric transit and wider current spread.[39] Myocardial injury has been documented after both high-voltage and low-voltage electric shock and has been attributed to the direct effects of current and coronary artery spasm.[39-41]

Cardiac and Respiratory Arrest

Cardiopulmonary arrest is the primary cause of immediate death due to electrical injury.[42] Ventricular fibrillation and other serious disturbances of the heart rhythm may occur as a direct result of electric shock. Respiratory arrest may occur secondary to

- Electric current passing through the brain and causing inhibition of respiratory center function
- Tetanic contraction of the diaphragm and chest wall musculature during current exposure
- Prolonged paralysis of respiratory muscles, which may continue for minutes after the shock current has terminated

If respiratory arrest persists, hypoxic cardiac arrest may occur.

Basic Life Support

Immediately after electrocution, respiration or circulation, or both, may fail. The patient may be apneic, mottled, unconscious, and in circulatory collapse from VF or asystole. The prognosis for recovery from electric shock is not readily predictable because the amplitude and duration of the charge usually are unknown. However, because many victims are young and without preexisting cardiopulmonary disease, they have a reasonable chance for survival, and vigorous resuscitative measures are indicated, even for those who appear dead on initial evaluation.

It is critically important that the rescuer be certain that rescue efforts will not put him or her in danger of electric shock. After the power is turned off by authorized personnel or the energized source is safely cleared from the victim, the rescuer should immediately determine the victim's cardiopulmonary status. If spontaneous respiration or circulation is absent, the BLS techniques outlined in this manual should be initiated.

As soon as possible, secure airway patency and provide ventilation and supplemental oxygen. When electric shock occurs in a location not readily accessible, such as on a utility pole, rescue breathing should be started at once, and the victim should be lowered to the ground as quickly as possible. Ventilations and chest compressions should be instituted immediately for victims with cardiac arrest.

Lightning Strike

Lightning strike, which accounts for more deaths than any other natural phenomenon, causes approximately 50 to 300 fatalities per year in the United States, with about twice that number sustaining serious injury.[43,44] Lightning injuries have a 30% death rate, and up to 70% of survivors sustain significant injury.[45]

The primary cause of death in lightning-strike victims is cardiac arrest, which may be due to primary VF or ventricular standstill (asystole).[46] Lightning acts as a massive direct-current countershock, depolarizing the entire myocardium at once and producing asystole. In many cases cardiac automaticity may restore organized cardiac activity, and the normal heart rhythm (sinus rhythm) may return spontaneously. However, concomitant respiratory arrest due to thoracic muscle spasm and suppression of the medullary respiratory center may continue after return of spontaneous circulation. Unless ventilatory assistance is provided, hypoxic cardiac arrest may occur.

Persons most likely to die of lightning injury if no treatment is forthcoming are those who suffer immediate cardiac arrest. Patients who have not suffered cardiac arrest already have an excellent chance of recovery because subsequent arrest is uncommon. Therefore, when multiple victims are struck simultaneously by lightning, usual triage priorities should be reversed. Rescuers should give highest priority to patients in cardiac or respiratory arrest.

For victims in cardiopulmonary arrest, BLS and ACLS should be instituted immediately. The goal is to oxygenate the heart and brain adequately until cardiac activity is restored. Victims with respiratory arrest may require only ventilation and oxygenation to avoid secondary hypoxic cardiac arrest. Resuscitative attempts may have higher success rates in lightning victims than in patients in whom cardiac arrest was due to other causes, and efforts may be effective even when the interval before the resuscitative attempt is prolonged.

Pregnancy

CPR of expectant mothers is unique because of dramatic alterations in maternal cardiovascular and respiratory function. During normal pregnancy, maternal cardiac output and blood volume increase up to 50%. Maternal heart rate, minute ventilation (ventilation per minute), and oxygen consumption also increase.[47] Together these changes render the pregnant woman more susceptible to and less tolerant of major cardiovascular and respiratory insults. Also, when the mother is supine, the pregnant uterus may compress the iliac vessels (major blood vessels to the lower body), the inferior vena cava, and the abdominal aorta, resulting in hypotension and as much as a 25% reduction in cardiac output.[48] Precipitating events for cardiac arrest during pregnancy include pulmonary embolism, trauma, hemorrhage of the placenta with consequent hypovolemia, amniotic fluid embolism, congenital and acquired cardiac disease, and complications of childbirth.

When cardiac arrest occurs in a pregnant woman, standard resuscitative measures and procedures can and should be taken without modification. If VF is present, it should be treated with defibrillation. If possible the heart rate of the fetus should be monitored and the defibrillator paddles placed somewhat (an interspace) higher than usual since the heart is usually pushed up.[49] If the fetal heart rate cannot be monitored but the mother is in VF, defibrillation must be performed immediately. Closed-chest compressions and support of ventilation should be done in accord with usual protocols. To minimize the effects of the pregnant uterus on venous return and cardiac output, a wedge, such as a pillow, should be placed under the right abdominal flank and hip to displace the uterus to the left side of the abdomen.[50] Alternatively, continuous manual displacement to the left may be used.

Allergies

Severe allergic reactions are rare, but when they occur, the consequences may be life-threatening. Exposure to a known allergen (foods, pollens, etc) or a reaction to an insect bite (eg, bee stings) may be the initial inciting event. Upper airway obstruction due to laryngeal edema or anaphylactic shock (life-threatening cardiovascular collapse) are the most severe consequences of an allergic reaction. Acting promptly when there is a strong suspicion of an allergic reaction can limit its adverse effects. After activating the EMS system, place the victim in a supine position and closely monitor the victim's airway. If respiratory or cardiac arrest occurs, initiate rescue breathing or CPR.

Asphyxiation

Asphyxiation (suffocation) is most commonly caused by inhaling a gas other than air or oxygen. It may occur during fires or from chemical spills or gas leaks. It can also be the result of breathing carbon monoxide in an enclosed space. The result is insufficient oxygen to the body, resulting in unconsciousness and ultimately cardiopulmonary arrest. Appropriate CPR should be performed.

Special Techniques and Pitfalls and Complications

If CPR is performed improperly or inadequately, chest compressions and rescue breathing may be ineffective in supporting life. Even properly performed CPR may result in complications.[51]

Rescue Breathing

The major problem associated with rescue breathing is gastric distention resulting from excess ventilation volume and rapid flow rates. Rescue breathing frequently causes gastric distention, especially in children. This distention can be minimized by maintaining an open airway and providing slow breaths only until visible chest rise is noted. Exceeding this level of chest rise can often result in gastric distention.

Marked distention of the stomach may promote regurgitation and reduce lung volume by elevating the diaphragm. If the stomach becomes distended during rescue breathing, recheck and reposition the airway, observe the rise and fall of the chest, and avoid excessive airway pressure by using slow ventilations. Continue slow rescue breathing without attempting to expel the stomach contents. Experience has shown that attempting to relieve stomach distention by manual pressure over the victim's upper abdomen is almost certain to cause regurgitation if the stomach is full. If regurgitation occurs spontaneously and no trauma is suspected, turn the victim's entire body to the side, wipe out the mouth, return the body to the supine position, and continue CPR.

Another concern of rescue (mouth-to-mouth) breathing is disease transmission. The Centers for Disease Control states that although it has not been shown that HIV is transmitted via saliva, the need for mouth-to-mouth resuscitation should be reduced as much as possible by making mouth-to-mask devices, resuscitation bags, or other ventilation devices available for use in areas in which the need for resuscitation is predictable.[52]

Use of the mouth-to-mask technique requires a transparent mask with a mouthpiece with a one-way valve. The clear mask permits the rescuer to see vomitus when it occurs. The one-way valve diverts the victim's exhaled gas away from the rescuer. The presence of an oxygen inlet allows the administration of supplemental oxygen during CPR. When available, the oxygen flow should be between 5 and 15 L/min.[53,54]

The user avoids direct contact with the victim's mouth, making assisted ventilation aesthetically more acceptable. However, the value of this technique in preventing transmission of infectious diseases is unknown. The cleaning/disinfecting of this device should be done in accordance with the manufacturer's guidelines.

Chest Compressions

Care should be taken to adhere to the recommendations for chest compression techniques. Pulselessness must be established before performing compressions. Proper CPR techniques lessen the possibility of complications.

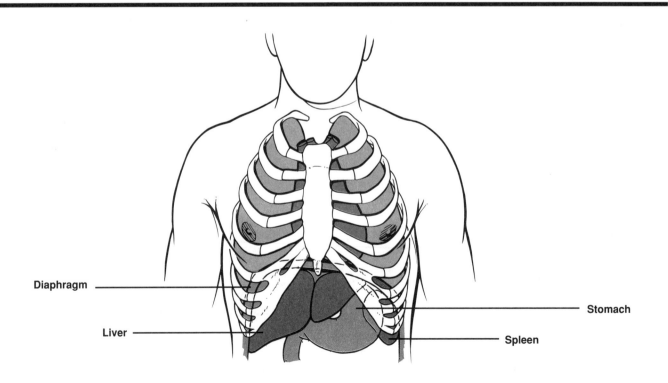

Fig 3. Intra-abdominal organs in relation to chest anatomy.

Even properly performed chest compressions can cause rib fractures in some patients. Other complications that may occur despite proper CPR techniques include fracture of the sternum, separation of the ribs from the sternum, pneumothorax, hemothorax, lung contusions, lacerations of the liver and spleen, and fat emboli. These complications may be minimized by careful attention to details of performance, but they cannot be prevented entirely. Accordingly, concern for injuries that may result even from properly performed CPR should not impede prompt and energetic application of the technique. The only alternative to timely initiation of effective CPR for the cardiac arrest victim is death.

Improper hand position for chest compressions should be avoided by careful identification of landmarks. Applying pressure too low on the chest may cause the tip of the sternum to cut into the liver and cause internal bleeding (Fig 3).

The rescuer's fingers should not rest on the victim's ribs during compression. Interlocking the fingers of the rescuer's hands may help avoid this. Pressure with fingers on the ribs or lateral (sideways) pressure increases the possibility of rib fractures and costochondral separations. Between compressions the heel of the hand must completely release its pressure but should remain in constant contact with the chest wall over the lower half of the sternum.

Compressions should be smooth, regular, and uninterrupted except for rescue breathing, patient reassessments, and defibrillation. There should be equal compression and relaxation cycles. Sudden or jerking movements should be avoided. Jabs can increase the possibility of injury to the ribs and internal organs and may decrease the amount of blood circulated by each compression. The lower half of the sternum of an adult must be depressed about 1 1/2 to 2 inches during each chest compression. Less depth of compression may be ineffective.

Summary. Complications and problems with effective administration of CPR can be lessened by adhering to the techniques and sequences described in chapters 4 and 6.

Unique Situations

Moving a Victim

Questions are often asked about managing CPR when it is necessary to change locations or to carry a victim up or down stairs.

Changing Location

A victim should not be moved for convenience from a cramped or busy location until effective CPR has been started and the victim has a spontaneous pulse or until help arrives so that CPR can be performed without interruption. If the location is unsafe, such as a burning building, the victim should be moved to a safe area and CPR then immediately started.

Stairways

In some instances a victim must be transported up or down a flight of stairs. It is best to perform CPR effectively at the head or foot of the stairs and to interrupt CPR at a predetermined signal and move as quickly as possible to the next level, where CPR should be resumed. Interruptions should be brief and must be avoided if possible.

Litters

CPR should not be interrupted while transferring a victim to an ambulance or other mobile emergency care unit. With a low-wheeled litter the rescuer can stand alongside, maintaining the locked-arm position for compression. With a high litter or bed the rescuer may have to kneel beside the victim on the bed or litter to gain the needed height over the victim's sternum.

CPR should not be interrupted unless endotracheal intubation is being performed by trained personnel or there are problems with transportation. If the rescuer is alone, a momentary delay of CPR may be necessary to activate the EMS system.[55]

References

1. *Heart and Stroke Facts: 1994 Statistical Supplement.* Dallas, Tex: American Heart Association; 1993.
2. North American Symptomatic Carotid Endarterectomy Trial Collaborators. Beneficial effect of carotid endarterectomy in symptomatic patients with high-grade carotid stenosis. *N Engl J Med.* 1991;325:445-453.
3. Antiplatelet Trialists' Collaboration. Secondary prevention of vascular disease by prolonged antiplatelet treatment. *Br Med J Clin Res.* 1988;296:320-331.
4. The Dutch TIA Trial Study Group. A comparison of two doses of aspirin (30 mg vs 283 mg a day) in patients after a transient ischemic attack or minor ischemic stroke. *N Engl J Med.* 1991; 325:1261-1266.
5. Hass WK, Easton JD, Adams HP Jr, et al. A randomized trial comparing ticlopidine hydrochloride with aspirin for the prevention of stroke in high-risk patients: Ticlopidine Aspirin Stroke Study Group. *N Engl J Med.* 1989;321:501-507.

6. Pickard JD, Murray GD, Illingworth R, et al. Effect of oral nimodipine on cerebral infarction and outcome after subarachnoid haemorrhage: British Aneurysm Nimodipine Trial. *Br Med J Clin Res.* 1989;298:636-642.

7. Broderick JP, Brott TG, Tomsick T, Barsan W, Spilker J. Ultra-early evaluation of intracerebral hemorrhage. *J Neurosurg.* 1990;72:195-199.

8. Kassell NF, Kongable GL, Torner JC, Adams HP Jr, Mazuz H. Delay in referral of patients with ruptured aneurysms to neurosurgical attention. *Stroke.* 1985;16:587-590.

9. Hijdra A, Vermeulen M, van Gijn J, van Crevel H. Respiratory arrest in subarachnoid hemorrhage. *Neurology.* 1984;34:1501-1503.

10. Di Pasquale G, Pinelli G, Andreoli A, Manini G, Grazi P, Tognetti F. Holter detection of cardiac arrhythmias in intracranial subarachnoid hemorrhage. *Am J Cardiol.* 1987;59:596-600.

11. Teasdale G, Jennett B. Assessment of coma and impaired consciousness: a practical scale. *Lancet.* 1974;2:81-84.

12. Schneider SM. Hypothermia: from recognition to rewarming. *Emerg Med Rep.* 1992;13:1-20.

13. Steinman AM. Cardiopulmonary resuscitation and hypothermia. *Circulation.* 1986;74(suppl IV):IV-29-IV-32.

14. Zell SC, Kurtz KJ. Severe exposure hypothermia: a resuscitation protocol. *Ann Emerg Med.* 1985;14:339-345.

15. Weinberg AD, Hamlet MP, Paturas JL, White RD, McAninch GW. *Cold Weather Emergencies: Principles of Patient Management.* Branford, Conn: American Medical Publishing Co; 1990:10-30.

16. Reuler JB. Hypothermia: pathophysiology, clinical settings, and management. *Ann Intern Med.* 1978;89:519-527.

17. Southwick FS, Dalglish PH Jr. Recovery after prolonged asystolic cardiac arrest in profound hypothermia: a case report and literature review. *JAMA.* 1980;243:1250-1253.

18. Woodhouse P, Keatinge WR, Coleshaw SR. Factors associated with hypothermia in patients admitted to a group of inner city hospitals. *Lancet.* 1989;2:1201-1205.

19. Danzl DF, Pozos RS, Auerbach PS, et al. Multicenter hypothermia survey. *Ann Emerg Med.* 1987;16:1042-1055.

20. Gallaher MM, Fleming DW, Berger LR, Sewell CM. Pedestrian and hypothermia deaths among Native Americans in New Mexico: between bar and home. *JAMA.* 1992;267:1345-1348.

21. Modell JH, Davis JH. Electrolyte changes in human drowning victims. *Anesthesiology.* 1969;30:414-420.

22. Modell JH, Davis JH. Is the Heimlich maneuver appropriate as first treatment for drowning? *Emerg Med Serv.* 1981;10:63-66.

23. Heimlich HJ. Subdiaphragmatic pressure to expel water from the lungs of drowning persons. *Ann Emerg Med.* 1981;10:476-480.

24. Patrick EA. A case report: the Heimlich maneuver. *Emergency.* 1981;13:45-47.

25. Heimlich HJ. The Heimlich maneuver: first treatment for drowning victims. *Emerg Med Serv.* 1981;10:58-61.

26. Quan L, Wentz KR, Gore EJ, Copass MK. Outcome and predictors of outcome in pediatric submersion victims receiving prehospital care in King County, Washington. *Pediatrics.* 1990;86:586-593.

27. Siebke H, Rod T, Breivik H, Link B. Survival after 40 minutes' submersion without cerebral sequelae. *Lancet.* 1975;1:1275-1277.

28. Bolte RG, Black PG, Bowers RS, Thorne JK, Corneli HM. The use of extracorporeal rewarming in a child submerged for 66 minutes. *JAMA.* 1988;260:377-379.

29. Copass MK, Oreskovich MR, Bladergroen MR, Carrico CJ. Prehospital cardiopulmonary resuscitation of the critically injured patient. *Am J Surg.* 1984;148:20-26.

30. Durham LA III, Richardson RJ, Wall MJ Jr, Pepe PE, Mattox KL. Emergency center thoracotomy: impact of prehospital resuscitation. *J Trauma.* 1992;32:775-779.

31. Pepe PE, Copass MK. Prehospital care. In: Moore EE, Ducker TB, American College of Surgeons, Committee on Trauma, eds. *Early Care of the Injured Patient.* 4th ed. Philadelphia, Pa: BC Decker; 1990:34-55.

32. Pepe PE. Emergency medical services systems and prehospital management of patients requiring critical care. In: Carlson R, Geheb M, eds. *Principles and Practice of Medical Intensive Care.* Philadelphia, Pa: WB Saunders Co; 1992, chap 1:9-24.

33. Browne BJ, Gaasch WR. Electrical injuries and lightning. *Emerg Med Clin North Am.* 1992;10:211-229.

34. Cooper MA. Electrical and lightning injuries. *Emerg Med Clin North Am.* 1984;2:489-501.

35. Kobernick M. Electrical injuries: pathophysiology and emergency management. *Ann Emerg Med.* 1982;11:633-638.

36. Budnick LD. Bathtub-related electrocutions in the United States, 1979 to 1982. *JAMA.* 1984;252:918-920.

37. Wallace JF. Electrical injuries. In: Wilson JD, Braunwald E, Isselbacher KJ, et al, eds. *Harrison's Principles of Internal Medicine.* 12th ed. New York, NY: McGraw-Hill Book Co, Health Professions Division; 1991:2202-2204.

38. Thompson JC, Ashwal S. Electrical injuries in children. *AJDC.* 1983;137:231-235.

39. Chandra NC, Siu CO, Munster AM. Clinical predictors of myocardial damage after high voltage electrical injury. *Crit Care Med.* 1990;18:293-297.

40. Ku CS, Lin SL, Hsu TL, Wang SP, Chang MS. Myocardial damage associated with electrical injury. *Am Heart J.* 1989;118:621-624.

41. Xenopoulos N, Movahed A, Hudson P, Reeves WC. Myocardial injury in electrocution. *Am Heart J.* 1991;122:1481-1484.

42. Homma S, Gillam LD, Weyman AE. Echocardiographic observations in survivors of acute electrical injury. *Chest.* 1990;97:103-105.

43. Epperly TD, Stewart JR. The physical effects of lightning injury. *J Fam Pract.* 1989;29:267-272.

44. Duclos PJ, Sanderson LM. An epidemiological description of lightning-related deaths in the United States. *Int J Epidemiol.* 1990;19:673-679.

45. Cooper MA. Lightning injuries: prognostic signs for death. *Ann Emerg Med.* 1980;9:134-138.

46. Kleiner JP, Wilkin JH. Cardiac effects of lightning stroke. *JAMA.* 1978;240:2757-2759.

47. Lee W, Cotton DB. Cardiorespiratory changes during pregnancy. In: Clark SL, Cotton DB, Hankins GDV, Phelan JP, eds. *Critical Care Obstetrics.* 2nd ed. Boston, Mass: Blackwell Scientific Publications; 1991:2-34.

48. Kerr MG. The mechanical effects of the gravid uterus in late pregnancy. *J Obstet Gynecol Br Commonw.* 1965;72:513-529.

49. Elkayan U, Gleicher N. Changes in cardiac findings during normal pregnancy. In: Elkayan U, Gleicher N, eds. *Cardiac Problems in Pregnancy.* 2nd ed. New York, NY: Alan R Liss Inc; 1990;31-38.

50. Rees GA, Willis BA. Resuscitation in late pregnancy. *Anaesthesia*. 1988;43:347-349.

51. Krischer JP, Fine EG, Davis JH, Nagel EL. Complications of cardiac resuscitation. *Chest*. 1987;92:287-291.

52. Centers for Disease Control. Recommendations for prevention of HIV transmission in health care settings. *MMWR*. 1987;36(suppl 2):1S-18S.

53. Hess D, Baran C. Ventilatory volumes using mouth-to-mouth, mouth-to-mask, and bag-valve-mask techniques. *Am J Emerg Med*. 1985;3:292-296.

54. Cummins RO, Austin D, Graves JR, Litwin PE, Pierce J. Ventilation skills of emergency medical technicians: a teaching challenge for emergency medicine. *Ann Emerg Med*. 1986;15:1187-1192.

55. Stults KR. Phone first. *J Emerg Med Serv*. 1987;12:28.

Pediatric Basic Life Support

Chapter 6

Cardiopulmonary resuscitation (CPR) and life support for infants and children should be part of a communitywide effort that integrates

- Education about injury prevention
- Pediatric basic life support (PBLS)
- Easy access to an EMS system sensitive to and prepared for the needs of children
- Pediatric advanced life support (ALS)
- Pediatric postresuscitation care

Out-of-hospital cardiopulmonary arrest is most likely to occur while children are under the supervision of parents or their surrogates.[1-5] BLS courses should therefore be offered to expectant parents, parents of young children, and others into whose care children are entrusted, such as day-care personnel, teachers, and sports supervisors. Many children who require resuscitation suffer from underlying conditions that predispose them to development of cardiopulmonary failure.[2] Parents of children at high risk— those with chronic diseases — should be particularly targeted for these courses. The content of BLS courses should emphasize preventive strategies, training in BLS techniques, and access to the EMS system. Although BLS requires no adjuncts, the healthcare provider should use adjuncts that are readily available, such as a barrier device and ventilation bag and mask, if the provider is trained in their use. Pediatric ALS courses should be mandatory for all prehospital and hospital personnel who care for infants and children.

Epidemiology

The epidemiology of pediatric cardiopulmonary arrest is different from that of adults. Sudden, primary cardiac arrest in young children is uncommon. Ventricular fibrillation has been reported in only 10% to 15% of children younger than 10 years who experience pulseless arrest outside of the hospital.[1,6-8] Ventricular tachycardia or fibrillation is more likely to be observed in older children (10 years or older), submersion victims, children with complex congenital heart disease, and children who arrest in the hospital.[7,8] More commonly, injury or disease causes respiratory or circulatory failure, which progresses to cardiopulmonary failure with hypoxemia and acidosis, culminating in asystolic or pulseless cardiac arrest.

Intact survival from prehospital normothermic *asystolic* or *pulseless* cardiac arrest in infants and children is uncommon. Survival averages 10% in most reports, and many of those who are resuscitated suffer permanent neurological damage.[2,6,7,9-12] The survival rate is slightly higher if ventricular fibrillation is present on the initial electrocardiogram.[7,8] In contrast, respiratory arrest alone is associated with a survival rate exceeding 50% when prompt resuscitation is provided, and most patients survive neurologically intact.[2,9,11] Aggressive prehospital BLS and ALS have also improved the outcome of drowning victims in pulseless cardiac arrest.[13,14] To improve the outcome of resuscitation in all children, vigorous prehospital resuscitation should be encouraged, with particular emphasis on providing effective ventilation and oxygenation and preventing cardiac arrest.

Pediatric cardiopulmonary arrest occurs most commonly at either end of the age spectrum — in children younger than 1 year and in adolescence. During infancy the most common causes of arrest are intentional and unintentional injury, apparent life-threatening events (including the condition formerly referred to as "near-miss" sudden infant death syndrome), respiratory diseases, airway obstruction (including foreign-body aspiration), submersion, sepsis, and neurological diseases.[2-6] Beyond infancy, injuries are the leading cause of pediatric prehospital cardiopulmonary arrest.[5,6,10,11]

Injury Prevention

Incidence

Injury is a leading cause of death in children and young adults and is responsible for more childhood deaths than all other causes combined.[15] Annually, pediatric injuries account for approximately 25 000 deaths, 600 000 hospital admissions, and 16 million emergency department visits, with direct costs exceeding $7.5 billion.[15-17] Injuries should be viewed as preventable.

The Science of Injury Control

Injury control attempts to prevent injury or to minimize its effects on the child and family. Injury control addresses preinjury, injury, and care of the injured patient. Examples of preinjury intervention include prevention of drunk driving and construction of barriers surrounding swimming pools. An intervention that may alter the consequence of injury is the use of restraining devices for children traveling in motor vehicles. Postinjury care of children must focus on public and professional education to ensure performance of optimal bystander CPR, skilled prehospital and hospital care, and effective rehabilitation.

In planning injury prevention strategies, three principles (based on the work of Haddon and others[18]) should be emphasized:

1. Passive injury prevention strategies, such as air bags or automatic seat and shoulder belts in cars, are generally more effective than active strategies that require repeated and conscious efforts.
2. Specific instructions are more likely to be followed than general advice.
3. Individual education, reinforced by community-wide educational programs, is more effective than isolated educational sessions.[18-20]

Epidemiology and Prevention of Common Childhood Injuries

Injury prevention programs will be most effective if they focus on injuries that are frequent and severe and for which proven prevention strategies are available. The six most common types of severe childhood injuries nationwide are motor vehicle passenger injuries, pedestrian injuries, bicycle injuries, submersion, burns, and firearm injuries.[15,16,21] Prevention of these would substantially reduce childhood deaths and disability.

Motor Vehicle Injuries

Motor vehicle–related trauma accounts for nearly half of all pediatric injuries and deaths.[15,21] Contributing factors include failure to use proper passenger restraints, inexperienced adolescent drivers, and alcohol abuse. Each of these factors should be addressed by injury prevention programs.

Proper use of child seat restraints and lap-shoulder harnesses can prevent an estimated 65% to 75% of serious injuries and fatalities to passengers under 4 years of age and 45% to 55% of all pediatric motor vehicle passenger injuries and deaths.[22] Use of proper seat restraints should be required and enforced by /law in every state and taught to parents of infants as well as to children during their early primary school

education. A 19-city National Highway Traffic Safety Administration (NHTSA) study documented that 20% of all child safety seats examined were seriously misused, and 1989-1990 estimates from voluntary screening programs have indicated that as many as 80% to 92% of child restraint devices in use are improperly installed.[23] Correct use of child restraint devices and safety belts must be taught and verified. Passive restraint devices, including adjustable shoulder harnesses and automatic lap and shoulder belts and air bags, should be further developed and implemented.

Adolescent drivers are responsible for a disproportionate number of motor vehicle–related injuries. Adolescent driver education classes *do not* reduce the incidence of collisions involving adolescent drivers. They have resulted in an increased number of licensed adolescent drivers without an improvement in safety.[24]

Adolescent drivers are inexperienced, and this inexperience, especially if coupled with alcohol, increases the risk of collision. Approximately 50% of adolescent motor vehicle fatalities involve alcohol.[22] In fact, a large proportion of all pediatric motor vehicle occupant deaths occur in vehicles operated by inebriated drivers.[25] Legislative and educational efforts must focus on elimination of drunk driving.

Pedestrian Injuries

Pedestrian injuries are a leading cause of death among children aged 5 to 9 years.[15,19] Injuries typically occur when a child darts out into the street and is struck by an automobile. Although promising educational programs attempt to improve the street-related behavior of children, roadway interventions such as adequate lighting, construction of sidewalks, and roadway barriers must also be pursued.

Bicycle Injuries

Every year approximately 200 000 children and adolescents are injured and more than 600 die from bicycle-related trauma.[15,16,21] Head injuries cause most bicycle-related morbidity and mortality, and bicycle-related trauma is a leading cause of severe pediatric closed-head injuries.[26] Use of bicycle helmets can prevent an estimated 85% of head injuries and 88% of brain injuries,[26] but many parents are unaware of the need for helmets, and children may be reluctant to wear them.[27] A successful bicycle helmet education program includes an ongoing communitywide multidisciplinary approach that provides focused information about the need for and effectiveness of helmets.

To be successful, such programs must ensure the acceptability, accessibility, and affordability of helmets.[16,27]

Submersion

Drowning is a significant cause of death and disability in children younger than 4 years and is the leading cause of death in this age group in several states.[15,19] For every death due to submersion, six children are hospitalized, and approximately 20% of hospitalized survivors suffer severe neurological sequelae.[15]

Parents should be aware of the dangers to children posed by any body of water. Young children and children with seizure disorders should never be left unattended in bathtubs or near swimming pools, ponds, or beaches. Drownings in swimming pools may be prevented if the pool is completely surrounded by a 5-foot fence with a self-closing, self-latching gate. The house *cannot* serve as a barrier to the pool if one of the house doors opens onto the pool area. Older children and adults who reside in homes with swimming pools should learn CPR, since prompt provision of BLS contributes to improved survival after submersion.[13,14] Children aged 5 years and older should know how to swim. No one should ever swim alone, and even supervised children should wear personal flotation devices when playing in rivers, streams, or lakes. Alcohol appears to be a significant risk factor in adolescent drowning. Hence control of alcohol and the use of personal flotation devices on waterways should be encouraged.

Burns

Approximately 80% of fire- and burn-related deaths result from house fires.[15,17] Most fire-related deaths occur in private residences,[28] usually in homes without working smoke detectors.[29] Smoke inhalation, scalds, and contact and electric burns are especially likely to affect children younger than 4 years. Socioeconomic factors such as overcrowding, single-parent families, scarce financial resources, inadequate child care, and distance from a fire department contribute to increased risk for burn injury.

Smoke detectors are one of the most effective interventions for prevention of deaths from burns and smoke inhalation. When used correctly, they can reduce the potential for death and severe injury by nearly 90%.[29] Parents should be aware of the effectiveness of these devices and the need to change smoke detector batteries twice every year.

Continued improvements in flammability standards for furniture, bedding, and home builders' materials should reduce the incidence of fire-related injuries and deaths. Child-resistant ignition products should also be explored. School-based fire-safety programs should be continued and evaluated.

Firearm Injuries

Firearms, particularly handguns, are responsible for an increasing number of unintentional pediatric injuries and an increasing number of pediatric homicides and suicides.[30] Annually more than 4500 children under 20 years of age die from firearm injuries, and thousands more are injured.[31] Firearm homicide is the leading cause of death among African-American adolescents and young adults and the second leading cause of death in all adolescent males.[31,32] The United States has the highest firearm-related homicide rate among young males of any industrialized nation, more than four times that of any other country.[31] The rising incidence of firearm injuries has paralleled the increased availability of handguns.[33] More than 66% of all homes in the United States contain firearms, and at least one home in every two contains handguns.[34] Thirty-four percent of surveyed high school students report easy access to guns, and an increasing number of children are carrying guns to school.[35-37] Most guns used in unintentional shootings are found in the home and are typically found loaded in readily accessible places.[34,38-41] The presence of a gun in the home has also been linked to an increased likelihood of adolescent suicide.[42]

Reduction in the incidence of firearm injuries requires removal of guns from each child's environment.[43] Every gun owner, potential gun purchaser, and parent must be made aware of the risks of firearms and the need to ensure that weapons are inaccessible to children.[43-45] Guns must be stored *only* in areas inaccessible to children. They should be stored unloaded, and ammunition should be stored in an area apart from the guns. The use of trigger locks should be encouraged and their efficacy determined. Owner liability laws and controlled distribution of handguns should be monitored for effectiveness. If such laws are found to be effective, their extension should be considered.

Prehospital Care

EMS systems were developed primarily for adults, and the requirements of pediatric victims have only recently been considered. Prehospital equipment is often inadequate to meet the needs of critically ill or injured infants and children, and prehospital personnel receive little pediatric emergency education. In EMS systems death rates are higher among children than adults, especially in areas where tertiary pediatric care is unavailable.[46-50] To overcome these deficiencies, communities should ensure that EMS personnel are trained and equipped to care for pediatric emergencies, that medical dispatchers have emergency protocols appropriate for children, and that emergency departments caring for children are appropriately staffed and equipped.[48-50] Emergency departments caring for acutely ill or injured children should have formal agreements with a pediatric tertiary service so that postresuscitation care for infants and children can be provided in a pediatric intensive care unit under the supervision of trained personnel.

The Sequence of Pediatric BLS: The ABCs of CPR and EMS Activation

Pediatric BLS includes sequential assessments and motor skills designed to support or restore effective ventilation and circulation to the child in respiratory or cardiorespiratory arrest. BLS can be performed by any trained bystander and is essential for the victim's eventual recovery. When cardiorespiratory arrest is present or impending, prompt access to advanced life support is also required.

Determine Responsiveness

The rescuer must quickly assess the presence or extent of injury and determine whether the child is conscious. The level of responsiveness is determined by tapping the child and speaking loudly to elicit a response. The victim should not be moved unnecessarily or shaken if spinal cord injury is suspected because such handling may aggravate the injury. If the child is unresponsive but breathing or struggling to breathe, the EMS system must be accessed so that the child can be rapidly transported to an advanced life support facility. Children with respiratory distress will often position themselves to maintain patency of a partially obstructed airway, and they should be allowed to remain in the position that is most comfortable for them.

Once unresponsiveness has been determined, the lone rescuer should shout for help and then provide BLS to the child, if necessary, for approximately 1 minute before the EMS system is activated. Since cardiac and cardiopulmonary arrest in children is most commonly associated with the development of hypoxemia rather than with ventricular arrhythmias, approximately 1 minute of rescue support may restore oxygenation

and effective ventilation or may prevent the child with respiratory arrest from developing cardiac arrest. If trauma has not occurred, the single rescuer may consider moving a small child close to a telephone so that the EMS system may be more easily called. The EMS medical dispatcher may then guide the rescuer through CPR. Movement of the child is mandatory if the child is found in a dangerous location (eg, in a burning building) or if CPR cannot be performed where the child is found (see also "Coordination of Compressions and Rescue Breathing" below). If a second rescuer is present during the initial assessment of the child, that rescuer should activate the EMS system as soon as the presence of cardiorespiratory distress is recognized.

A child should always be moved carefully, particularly if there is evidence of trauma. The likelihood of neck, spine, or bone injuries may be evident from the child's location and position. For example, traumatic injuries should be expected if a child is found unconscious at the side of the road or the base of a tree but will be unlikely if an unconscious infant is found in bed. If trauma is suspected, the cervical spine must be completely immobilized, and neck extension, flexion, and rotation must be prevented. When the child is moved, the head and body must be held and turned as a unit and the head and neck firmly supported so that the head does not roll, twist, or tilt.

Airway

Hypoxemia and respiratory arrest may cause or contribute to acute deterioration and cardiopulmonary arrest during childhood. Thus, establishment and maintenance of a patent airway and support of adequate ventilation are the most important components of BLS.

Assessment of Airway

Relaxation of muscles and passive posterior displacement of the tongue may lead to airway obstruction in the unconscious victim.[51] Whenever an unconscious, nonbreathing victim is found, the airway should be opened immediately. This is usually accomplished by the head tilt–chin lift maneuver. If neck injury is suspected, head tilt should be avoided and the airway opened by a jaw thrust while the cervical spine is completely immobilized. If the child is conscious and demonstrates spontaneous but labored respiratory efforts, time should not be wasted on an attempt to open the airway further. The child should instead be transported to an advanced life support facility as rapidly as possible.

Opening of Airway

Head Tilt–Chin Lift (Fig 1). To perform this technique:

- Place one hand on the child's forehead and tilt the head gently back into a neutral position. The neck is slightly extended.
- Place fingers, but not the thumb, of the other hand under the bony part of the lower jaw at the chin, and lift the mandible upward and outward.
- Be careful not to close the mouth or push on the soft tissues under the chin, because such maneuvers may obstruct rather than open the airway.
- If a foreign body or vomitus is visible, remove it.

Jaw Thrust. The jaw-thrust technique without head tilt is the safest method of opening the airway of the victim with suspected neck or cervical spine injury because it can be accomplished without extension of the neck.

- Place two or three fingers under each side of the lower jaw at its angle and lift the jaw upward and outward (Fig 2).

- If jaw thrust alone does not open the airway, slight head tilt may be added in patients with no evidence of cervical spine injury.
- If trauma is suspected and a second rescuer is present, that rescuer should immobilize the cervical spine (see "BLS in Trauma" below).

Breathing

Assessment of Breathing

After the airway is opened, the rescuer must determine if the child is breathing. The rescuer **looks** for a rise and fall of the chest and abdomen, **listens** for exhaled air, and **feels** for exhaled air flow at the mouth. If spontaneous breathing is present, a patent airway must be maintained. If the infant or child is unresponsive, has no evidence of trauma, and is obviously breathing effectively, the rescuer should place the victim in the **recovery position** and activate the EMS system. If the victim is breathing effectively and is small enough and is without evidence of trauma, the rescuer may carry the victim to the telephone to enable rapid activation of the EMS system.

To place the victim in the **recovery position:**

- Move the victim's head, shoulders, and torso simultaneously.
- Turn the victim onto his or her side.

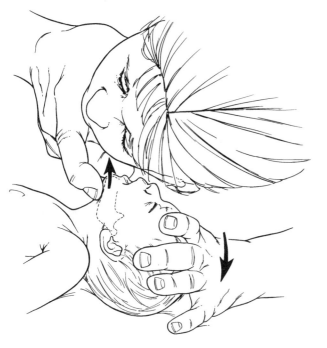

Fig 1. Opening the airway with the head tilt–chin lift maneuver. One hand is used to tilt the head, extending the neck. The index finger of the rescuer's other hand lifts the mandible outward by lifting on the chin. Head tilt should not be performed if cervical spine injury is suspected.

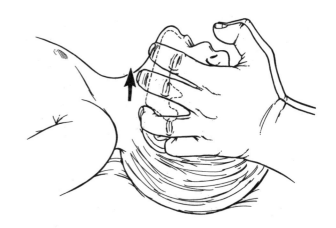

Fig 2. Opening the airway with the jaw-thrust maneuver. The airway is opened by lifting the angle of the mandible. The rescuer uses two or three fingers of each hand to lift the jaw while the remaining fingers guide the jaw upward and outward.

- The leg not in contact with the ground may be bent and the knee moved forward to stabilize the victim.
- Note that the victim should **not** be moved in any way if trauma is suspected and should not be placed in the recovery position if rescue breathing or CPR is required.

Rescue Breathing

If no spontaneous breathing is detected, rescue breathing must be provided while a patent airway is maintained by a chin lift or jaw thrust. If a mask with one-way valve or other infection control barrier is readily available, it should be used during rescue breathing. However, ventilation should not be delayed while such a device is located.

- First inhale deeply.
- *If the victim is an infant* (under 1 year old), place your mouth over the infant's nose and mouth, creating a seal (Fig 3).
- *If the victim is a large infant or a child* (1 to 8 years old), make a mouth-to-mouth seal and pinch the victim's nose tightly with the thumb and forefinger of the hand maintaining head tilt (Fig 4).
- Give two slow breaths (1 to 1½ seconds per breath) to the victim, pausing after the first breath to take a breath.

Pausing to take a breath maximizes oxygen content and minimizes carbon dioxide concentration in the delivered breaths.[52] If the rescuer fails to take this replenishing breath, the rescue breath will be low in oxygen and high in carbon dioxide.

Rescue breaths are the most important support for a nonbreathing infant or child. There is wide variation in the size of pediatric victims, so it is impossible to make precise recommendations about optimal pressure or volume of ventilations. The volume and pressure should be sufficient to cause the chest to rise. *If the child's chest does not rise during rescue breathing, ventilation is not effective.* The small airways of infants and children provide high resistance to airflow. To minimize the pressure required for ventilation and to prevent the development of gastric distention, breaths should be delivered slowly.[53] Slow delivery of breaths will allow delivery of an adequate volume of air and ensure effective lung and chest expansion. *The correct volume for each breath is the volume that causes the chest to rise.*

If air enters freely and the chest rises, the airway is clear. If air does not enter freely (if the chest does not rise), either the airway is obstructed or more breath volume or pressure is necessary. Since improper opening of the airway is the most common cause of airway obstruction, the rescuer should be prepared to reattempt opening of the airway and reattempt

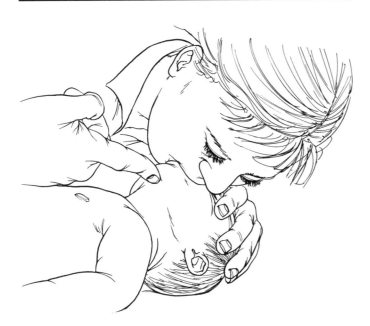

Fig 3. Rescue breathing in an infant. The rescuer's mouth covers the infant's nose and mouth, creating a seal. One hand performs head tilt while the other hand lifts the infant's jaw. Avoid head tilt if the infant has sustained head or neck trauma.

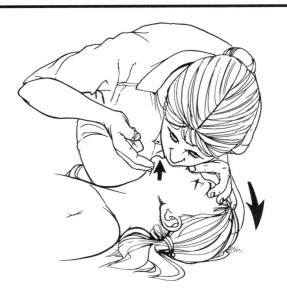

Fig 4. Rescue breathing in a child. The rescuer's mouth covers the mouth of the child, creating a mouth-to-mouth seal. One hand maintains head tilt; the thumb and forefinger of the same hand are used to pinch the child's nose. If head or neck trauma is suspected, immobilize the head in neutral position and *do not* perform head tilt.

ventilation if initial ventilation attempts are unsuccessful (ie, the chest does not rise). The victim's head will be placed in the neutral or sniffing position for the first attempt at ventilation. If ventilation is unsuccessful, the rescuer should move the victim's head into several positions of progressive neck extension, until a position of optimal airway patency results in effective rescue breathing (Fig 5). Such manipulation, however, should not be performed if neck or cervical spine trauma is suspected. Under these conditions airway opening should be provided by the jaw lift. If rescue breathing fails to produce chest expansion despite attempts at opening the airway, a foreign-body airway obstruction must be suspected (see "Foreign-Body Airway Obstruction" below).

Rescue breathing, especially if performed rapidly, may cause gastric distention.[54,55] Excessive gastric distention can, in turn, interfere with rescue breathing by elevating the diaphragm and thus compromise lung volume. Gastric distention may be minimized if rescue breaths are delivered slowly, since slow breaths will enable delivery of effective tidal volume at low inspiratory pressure. If two rescuers are present, the second rescuer may provide cricoid pressure to displace the trachea posteriorly, compressing the esophagus against the vertebral column. This maneuver may prevent gastric distention and reduce the likelihood of regurgitation. It cannot be performed by a single rescuer.

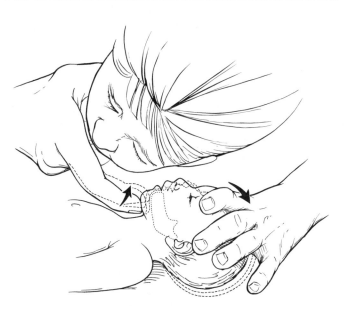

Fig 5. Movement of victim's head into positions of progressive neck extension until position of optimum airway patency (and effective ventilation) is achieved. Such manipulation of the head should *not* be performed if head, neck, or cervical spine injury is suspected.

Tracheostomy

Some pediatric victims, particularly those with chronic respiratory disease, may have a temporary tracheostomy tube in the trachea. Ventilation is provided through this tube. To prevent leakage of air when the rescuer blows into the tracheostomy tube, the victim's mouth and nose usually must be sealed by the rescuer's hand or by a tightly fitting face mask.

Mouth to Barrier Device

Some rescuers may prefer to use a barrier device during mouth-to-mouth ventilation. Many devices have been introduced, but few have been adequately studied. Two broad categories of devices are available: masks and face shields. Most masks have a one-way valve so that exhaled air does not enter the rescuer's mouth. Many face shields have no exhalation valve, and often air leaks around the shield. Barrier devices should ideally have a low resistance to gas flow to prevent rescuer fatigue. If rescue breathing is deemed necessary:

- Position the barrier device (face mask or face shield) over the victim's mouth and nose.
- Ensure an adequate air seal.
- Give slow inspiratory breaths (1 to 1½ seconds) as described above.

Further evaluation of the effectiveness of these devices is warranted. These devices are discussed in greater detail in chapter 4.

Circulation

Once the airway is opened and two rescue breaths have been provided, the rescuer determines the need for chest compression. The rescuer should be positioned beside the victim.

Assessment of Circulation: Pulse Check

If cardiac contractions are ineffective or absent, there will not be a palpable pulse in the central arteries. Two studies have documented the difficulty that laypersons have in locating peripheral pulses and counting the pulse rate in children.[56,57] If the child is not breathing spontaneously, heart rate and stroke volume are probably inadequate, so chest compressions are usually required. Complications associated with CPR (including cardiac compression) are uncommon in infants and children. Although rib fractures and injuries to the bony thorax have been observed following CPR in adults,[58] they have not been reported in infants[59] or children.[60] Thus the need for and validity of a pulse check by prehospital providers is questionable. Landmarks for locating pulses are provided here, but the lay rescuer should spend only a few seconds attempting to locate a pulse in a nonbreathing infant or child before providing chest compressions.

It is important to note that precordial activity represents an *impulse* rather than a pulse. The child's precordium may be quiet, and a precordial impulse may not be palpated despite the presence of satisfactory cardiac function and strong central pulse.[56] For this reason the apical impulse is not used in the pulse check.

Pulse Check in Infants. The short, chubby neck of infants under 1 year of age makes rapid location of the carotid artery difficult, so palpation of the *brachial artery* is recommended.[56] The femoral pulse is often palpated by healthcare professionals in a hospital setting. The brachial pulse is on the inside of the upper arm, between the infant's elbow and shoulder.

- With your thumb on the outside of the arm, gently press your index and middle fingers until you feel the pulse (Fig 6).

Pulse Check in Children. In children older than 1 year, the *carotid artery,* on the side of the neck, is the most accessible central artery to palpate. The carotid artery lies on the side of the neck between the trachea and the sternocleidomastoid muscles. To feel the artery:

- Locate the victim's thyroid cartilage (Adam's apple) with two or three fingers of one hand while maintaining head tilt with the other hand.

- Slide your fingers into the groove on the side of the neck closer to you, between the trachea and the sternocleidomastoid muscles.
- Gently palpate the artery (Fig 7).

If a pulse is present but spontaneous breathing is absent:

- Provide rescue breathing alone at a rate of 20 breaths per minute (once every 3 seconds) for the infant or the child until spontaneous breathing resumes.
- After giving approximately 20 breaths, activate the EMS system (see "Activation of the EMS System" below).

If a pulse is not palpable or heart rate is less than 60 *and* signs of poor systemic perfusion are present:

- Begin chest compressions.
- Coordinate compressions and ventilation.
- After providing approximately 20 cycles of compressions and ventilations, activate the EMS system.

Chest Compressions

Chest compressions are serial, rhythmic compressions of the chest that circulate oxygen-containing blood to the vital organs (heart, lungs, and brain) until advanced life support can be provided. Chest compressions must always be accompanied by ventilations.

The mechanism by which blood flow is circulated during chest compressions in pediatric victims remains controversial.[61-66] The thoracic pump theory suggests that blood circulates as a result of a change in

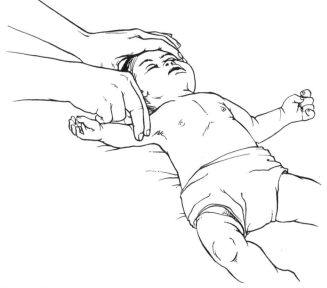

Fig 6. Palpating the brachial artery pulse in an infant.

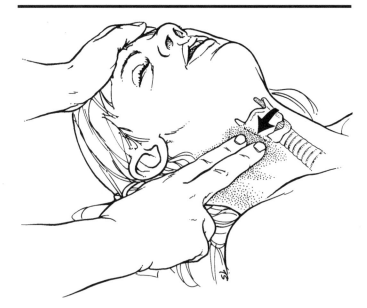

Fig 7. Locating and palpating the carotid artery pulse in the child.

intrathoracic versus extrathoracic pressures. According to the cardiac pump theory, circulation results from direct compression of the heart. In infants and perhaps in children, because of the greater mobility of the thoracic cage, direct heart compression may be an important mechanism of blood flow during compressions.[64]

To achieve optimal compressions:

• The child should be supine on a hard, flat surface.

For an infant the hard surface may be the rescuer's hand or forearm, with the palm supporting the infant's back (Fig 8, top). This maneuver effectively raises the infant's shoulders, allowing the head to tilt back slightly, into a position of airway patency.

If the infant is carried during CPR, the hard surface is created by the rescuer's forearm, which supports the length of the infant's torso, while the infant's head and neck are supported by the rescuer's hand. Care should be taken to keep the infant's head no higher than the rest of the body. The rescuer's other hand performs chest compression. The rescuer can lift the child to provide ventilation (Fig 8, bottom).

Chest Compression in the Infant. In infants the area of compression is the lower half of the sternum[67-69] (Fig 9). The technique for chest compression is as follows:

1. Use one hand to maintain the infant's head position (unless your hand is under the child's back). This may make it possible to ventilate without delaying to reposition the head.
2. Use your other hand to compress the chest. Place the index finger of that hand on the sternum just below the level of the infant's nipples. Place the middle fingers on the sternum, adjacent to the index finger. Sternal compression is performed approximately the width of one finger below the level of the nipples. Avoid compression of the xiphoid process, which is at the lowermost portion of the sternum, because such compression may injure the liver, stomach, or spleen.[70]
3. Using two or three fingers, compress the sternum approximately one third to one half the depth of the chest. This will correspond to a depth of about ½ to 1 inch, although these measurements are not precise.

   • The compression rate should be *at least* 100 times per minute.
   • Compressions must be coordinated with ventilations in a 5:1 ratio.

   With pauses for ventilation, the number of compressions will actually be at least 80 per minute.

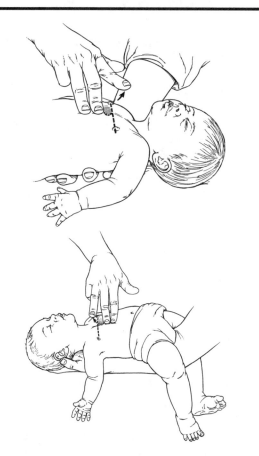

Fig 8. Cardiac compressions. Top, Infant supine on palm of the rescuer's hand. Bottom, Performing CPR while carrying the infant or small child. Note that the head is kept level with the torso. Compare Fig 9.

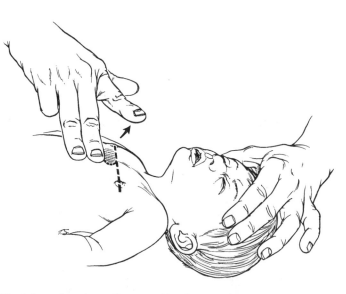

Fig 9. Locating proper finger position for chest compression in infant. Note that the rescuer's other hand is used to maintain head position to facilitate ventilation.

4. At the end of each compression, release pressure without removing the fingers from the chest. Allow the sternum to return briefly to its normal position. A smooth compression-relaxation rhythm without jerky movements should be developed, with equal time for compression and relaxation.
5. Activate the EMS system after you have provided approximately 1 minute of CPR (20 cycles).
6. If the victim resumes effective breathing, place the victim in the recovery position.

Chest Compression in the Child. Any child older than approximately 1 year up to 8 years is considered a child for the purposes of BLS. If the child is large or older than approximately 8 years, chest compression should be provided as described for adults.

1. Use one hand to maintain the child's head position so that it may be possible to ventilate without repositioning the head.
2. Using two fingers of the other hand, trace the lower margin of the victim's rib cage, on the side of the chest nearer you, to the notch where the ribs and sternum meet.
3. Note the location of the notch (where the ribs and sternum meet) and avoid compression over that notch, which includes the xiphoid.
4. Place the heel of your hand over the lower half of the sternum (between the nipple line and the notch), avoiding the xiphoid process. The long axis of the heel is over the long axis of the sternum (Fig 10).

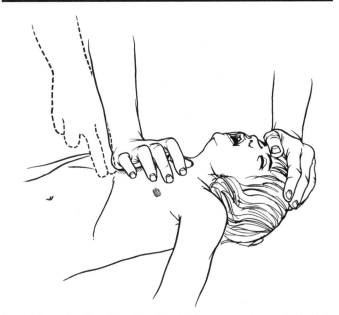

Fig 10. Locating hand position for chest compression in child. Note that the rescuer's other hand is used to maintain head position to facilitate ventilation.

5. Compress the chest to approximately one third to one half its total depth. This corresponds to a compression depth of about 1 to 1½ inches, but these measurements are not precise.

- The compression rate is 100 times per minute.
- Compressions must be coordinated with ventilation in a 5:1 compression-to-ventilation ratio.

With pauses for ventilation, the number of compressions will actually be approximately 80 compressions per minute.

6. The compressions should be smooth. Hold your fingers up off the ribs while the heel of your hand remains on the sternum. Allow the chest to return to its resting position after each compression, but do not lift your hand off the chest. Compression and relaxation should be of approximately equal duration.
7. Activate the EMS system after you have provided approximately 1 minute of CPR (20 cycles).
8. If the victim resumes effective breathing, place the victim in the recovery position.

Coordination of Compressions and Rescue Breathing

Chest compressions must always be accompanied by rescue breathing. At the end of every fifth compression, a pause of 1 to 1½ seconds should be allowed for a ventilation. The 5:1 compression-ventilation ratio for infants and children is used for both one and two rescuers. (The two-rescuer technique should be used only by healthcare providers.) The infant and child should be reassessed after 20 cycles of compressions and ventilations (approximately 1 minute, although this measurement is not precise) and every few minutes thereafter for any sign of resumption of spontaneous breathing or pulses.

Coordination of such rapid compressions and ventilations by a single rescuer may be difficult. Therefore, during cardiac compressions and between breaths for the infant, airway patency is maintained by head tilt using the hand that is not performing compression (Fig 9). Maintenance of head tilt in this way may reduce the time required to provide ventilation, enabling provision of an adequate number of compressions and ventilations every minute. Ventilation is adequate if effective chest expansion is observed with each breath provided by the rescuer. If the chest does not rise, the hand performing chest compressions should perform a chin lift to open the airway while ventilation is provided. That hand then returns to the compression position after ventilation.

In children, head tilt alone is often inadequate to maintain airway patency. Typically both hands are needed to perform the head tilt–chin lift maneuver with each ventilation. The time needed to position the hands for each breath, to locate landmarks, and to reposition the hand to perform compressions will reduce the total number of compressions provided. Therefore, when positioning the hand to perform chest compressions after ventilation, the rescuer should visualize the chest and return the hand to the approximate location used for the previous sequence of compressions. The full procedure to relocate the landmarks should not be performed each time a cycle of 5 compressions is begun.

A summary of BLS maneuvers in infants and children is presented in the Table. *Note:* Two-person CPR can be performed in children in a fashion similar to that for adults with appropriate changes in chest compressions and ventilations.

Activation of the EMS System

If the rescuer is alone, the EMS system should be activated after approximately 1 minute of rescue support (20 breaths including chest compressions, if necessary). If head and neck trauma are not present and the victim resumes spontaneous breathing, the rescuer should turn the unconscious victim to the side (recovery position) before leaving the victim to activate the EMS system. If head or neck trauma is suspected, the victim *should not* be turned.

If the victim is small and trauma is not suspected, it may be possible to carry the child (supporting the head and neck carefully) to a telephone while CPR is provided so that the EMS system can be activated. If the rescuer is unable to activate the EMS system, CPR should continue until help arrives or the rescuer becomes too exhausted to continue.

The rescuer calling the EMS system should be prepared to give the following information:

- The location of the emergency, including address and names of streets or landmarks
- The telephone number from which the call is being made
- What happened, eg, auto accident, drowning
- The number of victims
- The condition of the victim(s)
- The nature of the aid being given
- Any other information requested

The caller should hang up only after the dispatcher breaks the connection or if specifically instructed to do so by the dispatcher.

Foreign-Body Airway Obstruction

More than 90% of deaths from foreign-body aspiration in the pediatric age group occur in children younger than 5 years; 65% of the victims are infants.[71] With the development of consumer product safety standards regulating the minimum size of toys and toy parts for young children, the incidence of foreign-body aspiration has decreased. However, toys, balloons, or small objects and especially foods (eg, hot dogs, round candies, nuts, and grapes) may still be aspirated.[72, 73] Foreign-body airway obstruction should be suspected in infants and children who demonstrate the *sudden* onset of respiratory distress associated with coughing, gagging, stridor (a high-pitched, noisy sound), or wheezing.

Signs and symptoms of airway obstruction may also be caused by infections such as epiglottitis and croup, which produce airway edema. Infection should be suspected as the cause of airway obstruction if the child has a fever, particularly if accompanied by congestion, hoarseness, drooling, lethargy, or limpness. Children with an *infectious* cause of airway obstruction must be taken immediately to an emergency facility. Time should not be wasted in a futile and probably dangerous attempt to relieve this form of obstruction.

Attempts to clear the airway should be considered when foreign-body aspiration is witnessed or strongly suspected and when the airway remains obstructed (no chest expansion) during attempts to provide rescue breathing to the unconscious, nonbreathing infant or child. If foreign-body aspiration is witnessed or strongly suspected, the rescuer should encourage the child to continue spontaneous coughing and breathing efforts as long as the cough is forceful. Relief of airway obstruction should be attempted *only* if signs of *complete* airway obstruction are observed. These signs include ineffective cough (loss of sound), increased respiratory difficulty accompanied by stridor, development of cyanosis, and loss of consciousness. The EMS system should be activated as rapidly as possible by a second rescuer.

The Heimlich maneuver (subdiaphragmatic abdominal thrusts) is recommended for relief of complete upper airway obstruction in a child.[73,74] These thrusts increase intrathoracic pressure, creating an artificial cough that forces air and may force foreign bodies out of the airway. In the infant a combination of back blows and chest thrusts is recommended for relief of *complete* foreign-body airway obstruction. Although there is a paucity of data regarding relief of foreign-body airway obstruction in infants, existing scientific data do not suggest that back blows and chest thrusts are ineffective for this age group. Since the introduction of the first AHA BLS guidelines recommending back blows and chest thrusts, deaths due to foreign-body airway obstruction in infants and children aged 0 to 4 years have decreased by 60% from more than 450 per year to less than 170 per year.[71,73,75] There have been no scientific reports of complications from or failure of this technique when used in infants. Alternatively, rupture of the stomach, diaphragm, esophagus, and jejunum have been reported following the Heimlich technique.[76,77] Since the infant liver is large and unprotected by the rib cage, the risk of liver injuries may be high if the Heimlich maneuver were recommended for infants. Fatal liver lacerations in several infants have been linked to the application of sudden blunt abdominal trauma during child abuse.[78] For these reasons use of back blows and chest thrusts is recommended for relief of complete foreign-body airway obstruction in infants. Further data are needed to distinguish opinions and anecdotal experience from fact.

After maneuvers to relieve airway obstruction, the airway is opened using tongue-jaw lift. If the obstructing body is visible, it is removed. If no spontaneous breathing is observed, the airway is opened and rescue breathing is attempted. If the chest does not rise, the head is repositioned, the airway is opened, and rescue breathing is again attempted. If rescue breathing is still unsuccessful (ie, if the chest does not rise), maneuvers to relieve foreign-body obstruction should be repeated.

Manual Removal of Foreign Bodies

Blind finger sweeps should *not* be performed in infants and children since the foreign body may be pushed back into the airway, causing further obstruction. When the airway is opened in the *unconscious,* nonbreathing victim, the tongue-jaw lift is used.

- Grasp both the tongue and the lower jaw between the thumb and finger and lift (tongue-jaw lift). This action draws the tongue away from the back of the throat and may itself partially relieve the obstruction.
- If you see the foreign body, remove it.

The Infant: Back Blows and Chest Thrusts

The following sequence is used to clear a foreign-body obstruction from the airway of an infant. Back blows are delivered while the infant is supported in the prone position (face down) straddling the rescuer's forearm, with the head lower than the trunk. Chest thrusts

are delivered while the infant is supine, held on the rescuer's forearm, with the infant's head lower than the body. The rescuer should perform the following steps to relieve airway obstruction in the *conscious* infant:

1. Hold the infant face down, resting on the forearm. Support the infant's head by firmly holding the jaw. Rest your forearm on your thigh to support the infant. The infant's head should be lower than the trunk.
2. Deliver up to five back blows forcefully between the infant's shoulder blades, using the heel of the hand (Fig 11, top).

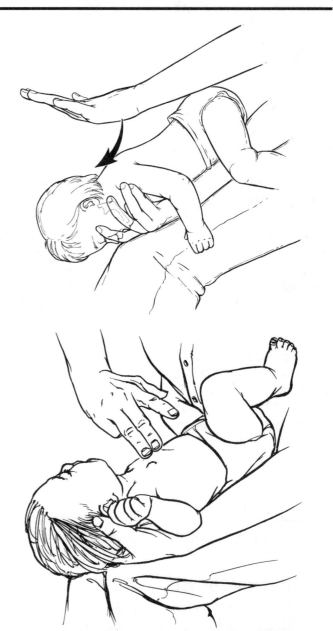

Fig 11. Back blows (top) and chest thrusts (bottom) to relieve foreign-body airway obstruction in the infant.

3. After delivering the back blows, place your free hand on the infant's back, holding the infant's head. The infant is effectively sandwiched between your two hands and arms. One hand supports the head and neck, jaw, and chest while the other supports the back.
4. Turn the infant while the head and neck are carefully supported, and hold the infant in the supine position, draped on the thigh. The infant's head should remain lower than the trunk.
5. Give up to five quick downward chest thrusts in the same location and manner as chest compressions — two fingers placed on the lower half of the sternum, approximately one finger's breadth below the nipples (Fig 11, bottom).

If the rescuer's hands are small or the infant is large, these maneuvers may be hard to perform. If so, place the infant supine on the lap, with the head lower than the trunk and the head firmly supported. After you have given up to five back blows, turn the infant as a unit to the supine position and give up to five chest thrusts.

Steps 1 through 5 should be repeated until the object is expelled or the infant loses consciousness. If the infant loses consciousness, open the airway using a tongue-jaw lift and remove the foreign object if you see it and attempt rescue breathing and relief of airway obstruction.

If the victim is or becomes unconscious:

1. Open the infant's airway. If the loss of consciousness is witnessed and foreign-body obstruction is suspected, lift the chin using a tongue-jaw lift and if you see a foreign object, remove it with a finger sweep.
2. Attempt rescue breathing.
3. If the first attempt is unsuccessful, reposition the head and reattempt ventilation.
4. If ventilation is unsuccessful, give five back blows and five chest thrusts.
5. Open the mouth using a tongue-jaw lift and remove the foreign object if you see it.
6. Repeat steps 2 through 4 until ventilation is successful (the chest rises).
7. Activate the EMS system after approximately 1 minute, then resume efforts.
8. If the victim resumes effective breathing, place in the recovery position and monitor closely until rescue personnel arrive.

The Child: The Heimlich Maneuver

Abdominal Thrusts With Victim Conscious (Standing or Sitting)

Perform the following steps to relieve complete airway obstruction in the *conscious* victim:

1. Stand behind the victim, arms directly under the victim's axillae encircling the victim's torso.
2. Place the thumb side of one fist against the victim's abdomen in the midline slightly above the navel and well below the tip of the xiphoid process.
3. Grasp the fist with the other hand and exert a series of quick upward thrusts (Fig 12). Do not touch the xiphoid process or the lower margins of the rib cage because force applied to these structures may damage internal organs.
4. Each thrust should be a separate, distinct movement, intended to relieve the obstruction. Continue abdominal thrusts until the foreign body is expelled or the patient loses consciousness.
5. If the victim loses consciousness, open the airway using a tongue-jaw lift and if you see the obstructing object, remove it with a finger sweep.
6. Attempt rescue breathing. If the chest fails to rise, reposition the head and reattempt rescue breathing again. If the airway remains obstructed in the unconscious victim, repeat the Heimlich maneuver (see below).

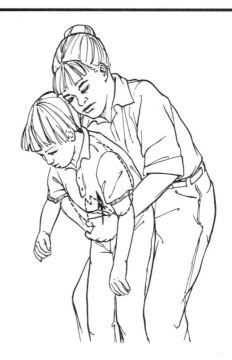

Fig 12. Abdominal thrusts with victim standing or sitting (conscious).

Abdominal Thrusts for the Victim Who Is Unconscious or Who Becomes Unconscious

The rescuer should perform the following steps:

1. Place the victim supine.
2. If the loss of consciousness is witnessed and foreign-body airway obstruction is suspected, open the airway using a tongue-jaw lift and remove the object with a finger sweep if you see it.
3. Attempt rescue breathing. If ventilation is unsuccessful, reposition the head and reattempt ventilation. If ventilation is still unsuccessful, continue with steps 4 through 8 below.
4. Kneel beside the victim or straddle the victim's hips.
5. Place the heel of one hand on the child's abdomen in the midline slightly above the navel and well below the rib cage and xiphoid process. Place the other hand on top of the first.
6. Press both hands into the abdomen with a quick upward thrust (Fig 13). Each thrust is directed upward in the midline and should not be directed to either side of the abdomen. Perform a series of five thrusts. Each thrust should be a separate and distinct movement.
7. Open the airway by grasping both the tongue and lower jaw and lifting the mandible (tongue-jaw lift). If you see the foreign body, remove it using a finger sweep.
8. Repeat steps 3 through 7 until ventilation is successful.

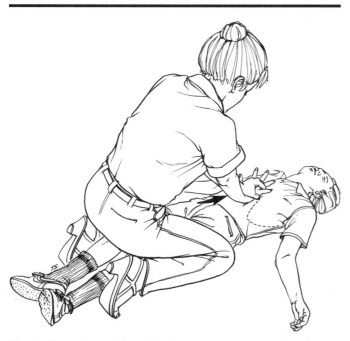

Fig 13. Abdominal thrusts with victim lying (conscious or unconscious).

Summary of BLS Maneuvers in Infants and Children

Maneuver	Infant (<1 y)	Child (1 to 8 y)
Airway	Head tilt–chin lift (if trauma is present, use jaw thrust)	Head tilt–chin lift (if trauma is present, use jaw thrust)
Breathing		
Initial	Two breaths at 1 to 1½ s/breath	Two breaths at 1 to 1½ s/breath
Subsequent	20 breaths/min (approximate)	20 breaths/min (approximate)
Circulation		
Pulse check	Brachial/femoral	Carotid
Compression area	Lower half of sternum	Lower half of sternum
Compression width	2 or 3 fingers	Heel of 1 hand
Depth	Approximately one third to one half the depth of the chest	Approximately one third to one half the depth of the chest
Rate	At least 100/min	100/min
Compression-ventilation ratio	5:1 (pause for ventilation)	5:1 (pause for ventilation)
Foreign-body airway obstruction	Back blows/chest thrusts	Heimlich maneuver

BLS in Trauma

Prompt assessment and intervention are essential for successful treatment of childhood trauma. Resuscitation should begin as soon as possible after injury, preferably at the scene. Improper resuscitation and failure to adequately open and maintain the airway have been identified as major causes of preventable trauma death.[79]

The pediatric trauma victim requires meticulous support of airway, breathing, and circulation. The child's small airways may become obstructed by soft tissue swelling, blood, vomitus, or dental fragments, so these causes of airway obstruction should be anticipated. Whenever head or neck injury is suspected, the cervical spine must be completely immobilized when the airway is opened. This is best accomplished by a combined jaw-thrust and spinal stabilization maneuver, using only the amount of manual control necessary to prevent cranial-cervical motion[80] (Fig 14). The head tilt–chin lift is contraindicated in trauma victims because it may worsen existing cervical spinal injury.

Care must be taken to ensure that the neck is maintained in a neutral position because the prominent occiput of the child predisposes the neck to slight flexion when the child is placed on a flat surface.[81]

If two rescuers are present, the first rescuer opens the airway with a jaw-thrust maneuver while the second rescuer ensures that the cervical spine is absolutely immobilized in a neutral position. Traction on or movement of the neck must be avoided because it may result in conversion of a partial spinal cord injury to a complete injury. Once the airway is controlled, the cervical spine should be immobilized using a semirigid cervical collar and a spine board, linen rolls, and tape, and oxygenation and ventilation should be supported.[82]

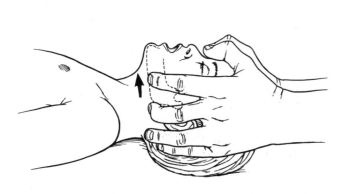

Fig 14. Combined jaw thrust–spine stabilization maneuver for the pediatric trauma victim.

References

1. Walsh CK, Krongrad E. Terminal cardiac electrical activity in pediatric patients. *Am J Cardiol.* 1983;51:557-561.

2. Zaritsky A, Nadkarni V, Getson P, Kuehl K. CPR in children. *Ann Emerg Med.* 1987;16:1107-1111.

3. Friesen RM, Duncan P, Tweed WA, Bristow G. Appraisal of pediatric cardiopulmonary resuscitation. *Can Med Assoc J.* 1982;126:1055-1058.

4. Torphy DE, Minter MG, Thompson BM. Cardiorespiratory arrest and resuscitation of children. *Am J Dis Child.* 1984;138:1099-1102.

5. Gausche M, Seidel JS, Henderson DP, et al. Pediatric deaths and emergency medical services (EMS) in urban and rural areas. *Pediatr Emerg Care.* 1989;5:158-162.

6. Eisenberg M, Bergner L, Hallstrom A. Epidemiology of cardiac arrest and resuscitation in children. *Ann Emerg Med.* 1983; 12:672-674.

7. Coffing CR, Quan L, Graves JR, et al. Etiologies and outcomes of the pulseless, nonbreathing pediatric patient presenting with ventricular fibrillation. *Ann Emerg Med.* 1992; 21:1046. Abstract.

8. Gillis J, Dickson D, Rieder M, Steward D, Edmonds J. Results of inpatient pediatric resuscitation. *Crit Care Med.* 1986; 14:469-471.

9. Lewis JK, Minter MG, Eshelman SJ, Witte MK. Outcome of pediatric resuscitation. *Ann Emerg Med.* 1983;12:297-299.

10. O'Rourke PP. Outcome of children who are apneic and pulseless in the emergency room. *Crit Care Med.* 1986;14:466-468.

11. Schoenfeld PS, Baker MD. Management of cardiopulmonary and trauma resuscitation in the pediatric emergency department. *Pediatrics.* 1993; 91:726-729.

12. Hazinski MF, Chahine AA, Holcomb GW III, Morris JA Jr. Outcome of cardiovascular collapse in pediatric blunt trauma. *Ann Emerg Med.* In press.

13. Quan L, Wentz KR, Gore EJ, Copass MK. Outcome and predictors of outcome in pediatric submersion victims receiving prehospital care in King County, Washington. *Pediatrics.* 1990;86:586-593.

14. Kyriacou DN, Kraus JF, Arcinue E. Effect of immediate resuscitation on childhood outcomes after aquatic submersion injury. *Ann Emerg Med.* 1992; 21:1046. Abstract.

15. Division of Injury Control, Center for Environmental Health and Injury Control, Centers for Disease Control. Childhood injuries in the United States. *Am J Dis Child.* 1990;144:627-646.

16. DiGuiseppi CG, Rivara FP, Koepsell TD, Polissar L. Bicycle helmet use by children: evaluation of a community-wide helmet campaign. *JAMA.* 1989;262:2256-2261.

17. Rice DP, Mackenzie EJ, and Associates. *Cost of Injury in the United States: A Report to Congress.* Atlanta, Ga: Division of Injury, Epidemiology, and Control, Center for Environmental Health and Injury Control, Centers for Disease Control; 1989.

18. Haddon W, Suchman EA, Klein O. *Accident Research: Methods and Approaches.* New York, NY: Harper and Row; 1964.

19. Guyer B, Ellers B. Childhood injuries in the United States: mortality, morbidity, and cost. *Am J Dis Child.* 1990;144: 649-652.

20. Cushman R, James W, Waclawik H. Physicians promoting bicycle helmets for children: a randomized trial. *Am J Public Health.* 1991;81:1044-1046.

21. Centers for Disease Control. Fatal injuries to children—United States, 1986. *JAMA.* 1990;264:952-953.

22. The National Committee for Injury Prevention and Control. Traffic injuries. In: *Injury Prevention: Meeting the Challenge. Am J Prev Med.* 1989;5(suppl):115-144.

23. Safety Belt USA: Unpublished reports, Virginia Commonwealth University, Transportation Center. 1990.

24. Robertson LS. Crash involvement of teenaged drivers when driver education is eliminated from high school. *Am J Public Health.* 1980;70:599-603.

25. Margolis LH, Kotch J, Lacey JH. Children in alcohol-related motor vehicle crashes. *Pediatrics.* 1986;77:870-872.

26. Thompson RS, Rivara FP, Thompson DC. A case-control study of the effectiveness of bicycle safety helmets. *N Engl J Med.* 1989;320:1361-1367.

27. DiGuiseppi CG, Rivara FP, Koepsell TD. Attitudes toward bicycle helmet ownership and use by school-age children. *Am J Dis Child.* 1990;144:83-86.

28. The National Committee for Injury Prevention and Control. Residential injuries. In: *Injury Prevention: Meeting the Challenge. Am J Prev Med.* 1989;5(suppl):153-162.

29. *An Evaluation of Residential Smoke Detector Performance Under Actual Field Conditions.* Washington, DC: Federal Emergency Management Agency; 1980.

30. *Facts About Kids and Handguns.* Washington, DC: Center to Prevent Handgun Violence; May 1990.

31. Fingerhut LA, Kleinman JC, Godfrey E, Rosenberg H. Firearm mortality among children, youth and young adults, 1-34 years of age, trends and current status: United States, 1979-1988. *Monthly Vital Stat Rep.* 1991;39:1-16. No. 11.

32. Fingerhut LA, Ingram DD, Feldman JJ. Firearm homicide among black teenage males in metropolitan counties: comparison of death rates in two periods, 1983 through 1985 and 1987 through 1989. *JAMA.* 1992;267:3054-3058.

33. Wintemute GJ. Firearms as a cause of death in the United States, 1920-1982. *J Trauma.* 1987;27:532-536.

34. Weil DS, Hemenway D. Loaded guns in the home: analysis of national random survey of gun owners. *JAMA.* 1992;267:3033-3037.

35. *Caught in the Crossfire: A Report on Gun Violence in Our Nation's Schools.* Washington, DC: Center to Prevent Handgun Violence; September 1990.

36. Callahan CM, Rivara FP. Urban high school youth and handguns: a school-based survey. *JAMA.* 1992;267:3038-3042.

37. Weapon-carrying among high-school students: United States, 1990. *MMWR.* 1991;40:681-684.

38. Wintemute GJ, Teret SP, Kraus JF, Wright MA, Bradfield G. When children shoot children: 88 unintended deaths in California. *JAMA.* 1987;257:3107-3109.

39. *Child's Play: A Study of 266 Unintentional Handgun Shootings of Children.* Washington, DC: Center to Prevent Handgun Violence; 1990.

40. *The Killing Seasons: A Study of When Unintentional Handgun Shootings Among Children Occur.* Washington, DC: Center to Prevent Handgun Violence; 1990.

41. Beaver BL, Moore VL, Peclet M, Haller JA Jr, Smialek J, Hill JL. Characteristics of pediatric firearm fatalities. *J Pediatr Surg.* 1990;25:97-99.

42. Brent DA, Perper JA, Allman CJ, Mortiz GM, Wartella ME, Zelenak JP. The presence and accessibility of firearms in the homes of adolescent suicides: a case-control study. *JAMA.* 1991;266:2989-2995.

43. Christoffel KK. Toward reducing pediatric injuries from firearms: charting a legislative and regulatory course. *Pediatrics.* 1991;88:294-305.

44. American Academy of Pediatrics Committee on Injury and Poison Prevention. Policy statement: firearm injuries affecting the pediatric population. *AAP News.* 1992;8:22-33.

45. Christoffel KK. Pediatric firearm injuries: time to target a growing population. *Pediatr Ann.* 1992;21:430-436.

46. Seidel JS. Emergency medical services and the pediatric patient: are the needs being met? II: training and equipping emergency service providers for pediatric emergencies. *Pediatrics.* 1986;78:808-812.

47. Applebaum D. Advanced prehospital care for pediatric emergencies. *Ann Emerg Med.* 1985;14:656-659.

48. Seidel JS. EMS-C in urban and rural areas: the California experience. In: Haller JA Jr, ed. *Emergency Medical Services for Children: Report of the 97th Ross Conference on Pediatric Research.* Columbus, Ohio: Ross Laboratories; 1989:22-30.

49. Seidel JS, Henderson DP, eds. *Emergency Medical Services for Children: A Report to the Nation.* Washington DC: National Center for Education in Maternal and Child Health; 1991.

50. Durch JS, Lohr KN, eds. *Emergency Medical Services for Children.* Washington, DC: National Academy Press; 1993.

51. Ruben HM, Elam JO, Ruben AM, Greene DG. Investigation of upper airway problems in resuscitation, I: studies of pharyngeal x-rays and performance by laymen. *Anesthesiology.* 1961;22:271-279.

52. Tendrup TE, Kanter RK, Cherry RA. A comparison of infant ventilation methods performed by prehospital personnel. *Ann Emerg Med.* 1989;18:607-611.

53. Melker R, Cavallaro D, Krischer J. One rescuer CPR — a reappraisal of present recommendations for ventilation. *Crit Care Med.* 1981;9:423.

54. Melker RJ. Asynchronous and other alternative methods of ventilation during CPR. *Ann Emerg Med.* 1984;13(pt 2):758-761.

55. Melker RJ, Banner MJ. Ventilation during CPR: two-rescuer standards reappraised. *Ann Emerg Med.* 1985;14:397-402.

56. Cavallaro DL, Melker RJ. Comparison of two techniques for detecting cardiac activity in infants. *Crit Care Med.* 1983;11:189-190.

57. Lee CJ, Bullock LJ. Determining the pulse for infant CPR: time for a change? *Milit Med.* 1991;156:190-199.

58. Nagel EL, Fine EG, Krischer JP, Davis JH. Complications of CPR. *Crit Care Med.* 1981;9:424.

59. Spevak MR, Kleinman PK, Belanger PL, Richmond MD. Does cardiopulmonary resuscitation cause rib fractures in infants? Postmortem radiologic-pathologic study. *Radiology.* 1990;177P:162. Abstract. (National Program, RSNA '90)

60. Feldman KW, Brewer DK. Child abuse, cardiopulmonary resuscitation, and rib fractures. *Pediatrics.* 1984;73:339-342.

61. Zaritsky A. Selected concepts and controversies in pediatric cardiopulmonary resuscitation. *Crit Care Clin.* 1988;4:735-754.

62. Berkowitz ID, Chantarojanasiri T, Koehler RC, et al. Blood flow during cardiopulmonary resuscitation with simultaneous compression and ventilation in infant pigs. *Pediatr Res.* 1989;26:558-564.

63. Krischer JP, Fine EG, Weisfeldt ML, Guerci AD, Nagel E, Chandra N. Comparison of prehospital conventional and simultaneous compression-ventilation cardiopulmonary resuscitation. *Crit Care Med.* 1989;17:1263-1269.

64. Dean JM, Koehler RC, Schleien CL, et al. Age-related changes in chest geometry during cardiopulmonary resuscitation. *J Appl Physiol.* 1987;62:2212-2219.

65. Dean JM, Koehler RC, Schleien CL, Atchison D, et al. Improved blood flow during prolonged cardiopulmonary resuscitation with 30% duty cycle in infant pigs. *Circulation.* 1991;84:896-904.

66. Deshmukh HG, Weil MH, Gudipati CV, Trevino RP, Bisera J, Rackow EC. Mechanism of blood flow generated by precordial compression during CPR, I: studies on closed-chest precordial compression. *Chest.* 1989;95:1092-1099.

67. Finholt DA, Kettrick RG, Wagner HR, Swedlow DB. The heart is under the lower third of the sternum: implications for external cardiac massage. *Am J Dis Child.* 1986;140:646-649.

68. Phillips GW, Zideman DA. Relation of infant heart to sternum: its significance in cardiopulmonary resuscitation. *Lancet.* 1986;1:1024-1025.

69. Orlowski JP. Optimal position for external cardiac massage in infants and children. *Crit Care Med.* 1984;12:224.

70. Thaler MM, Krause VW. Serious trauma in children after external cardiac massage. *N Engl J Med.* 1962;267:500-501.

71. National Safety Council. How people died accidentally in 1983. In: *Accident Facts 1984.* Chicago, Ill: National Safety Council; 1984.

72. Harris CS, Baker SP, Smith GA, Harris RM. Childhood asphyxiation by food: a national analysis and overview. *JAMA.* 1984;251:2231-2235.

73. Reilly JS. Prevention of aspiration in infants and young children: federal regulations. *Ann Otol Rhinol Laryngol.* 1990;99:273-276.

74. Heimlich HJ. A life-saving maneuver to prevent food-choking. *JAMA.* 1975;234:398-401.

75. National Safety Council. How people died in home accidents: 1978. In: *Accident Facts 1979.* Chicago, Ill: National Safety Council; 1979:81-82.

76. Fink JA, Klein RL. Complications of the Heimlich maneuver. *J Pediatr Surg.* 1989;24:486-487.

77. Van der Ham AC, Lange JF. Traumatic rupture of the stomach after Heimlich maneuver. *J Emerg Med.* 1990;8:713-715.

78. Cooper A, Floyd T, Barlow B, et al. Major blunt abdominal trauma due to child abuse. *J Trauma.* 1988;28:1483-1487.

79. Dykes EH, Spence LJ, Young JG, Bohn DJ, Filler RM, Wesson DE. Preventable pediatric trauma deaths in a metropolitan region. *J Pediatr Surg.* 1989;24:107-110.

80. Cooper A, Foltin G, Tunik M. Airway control in the unconscious child victim: description of a new maneuver. *Ped Emerg Care.* In press.

81. Herzenberg JE, Hensinger RN, Dedrick DK, Phillips WA. Emergency transport and positioning of young children who have an injury of the cervical spine: the standard backboard may be hazardous. *J Bone Joint Surg Am.* 1989;71:15-22.

82. Soud T, Pieper P, Hazinski MF. Pediatric trauma. In: Hazinski MF, ed. *Nursing Care of the Critically Ill Child.* 2nd ed. St Louis, Mo: CV Mosby Co; 1992:842-843.

Ethical and Legal Considerations

The goal of medical therapy is to preserve life, restore health, relieve suffering, and limit disability. These goals are influenced by society's common values — autonomy, beneficence, and justice. CPR is a medical therapy that must be considered within the context of these goals and ethical values. It should be used to preserve life, restore health, and limit disability. Often these goals cannot be achieved. CPR, like all medical interventions, should be considered to have indications and contraindications to its use. Ethical values should be considered, including the potential benefit to patients and patients' requests regarding its use. CPR is unique, however, in that there is no time for deliberation before beginning resuscitation, and unlike other medical therapies, CPR is instituted without physician orders. It is begun on the premise of implied consent. Because one of the primary goals of medical therapy is to preserve life, there is a strong presumption for the institution of CPR, and the standard of care remains that CPR should be initiated promptly except in specific circumstances. The purpose of this chapter is to guide healthcare providers in making difficult decisions about starting and stopping CPR. These are guidelines only. Each decision must be individualized and made with compassion and reason.[1]

Values in Decision Making

Beneficence and advocacy are values encouraging the healthcare provider to defend the individual patient's best interest. Sometimes there is disagreement between the physician's view and the patient's view of what is in the patient's best interest, and this should be resolved in favor of the patient's view where possible. Patient autonomy has become a dominant value in medical decision making. A competent and informed person has a moral right to choose whether to consent to or to refuse medical interventions.[2] The physician has an obligation to determine the patient's decision-making capacity and to provide him or her with enough information to make an informed decision. If the patient cannot make an informed decision about CPR, the attending physician should consider the patient's advance directives or decisions by appropriate surrogates as well as the likely response to CPR.

By using advance directives, competent patients indicate what interventions they wish to refuse or accept should they lose the capacity to make decisions about their care. Advance directives include conversations, written directives, living wills, and durable powers of attorney for health care. Advance directives are often vague and require interpretation and the development of a care plan with specific physician orders (ie, No CPR). Physicians should endeavor to have all patients clearly state their advance directives, irrespective of their health status.

The term *No CPR* is used to convey the meaning that, in the event of a cardiac arrest, no cardiopulmonary resuscitative measures will be instituted. The No-CPR order provides that if the patient is in cardiac arrest, no further treatment will be provided. It does not preclude the administration of other forms of beneficial medical therapy (eg, oxygen, IV fluids), nor does it preclude resuscitative efforts before cardiac arrest.[3] In some communities the terms *DNR* (Do Not Resuscitate) or *DNAR* (Do Not Attempt Resuscitation) are used to withhold CPR.

The physician must obtain informed consent for writing a No-CPR order or provide informed disclosure in cases where it can be demonstrated that CPR is of no physiological benefit.[4]

The right to refuse care does not mean that the patient has the right to demand nonbeneficial treatments. However, it is often difficult to determine if a resuscitative attempt is futile or of no benefit to the patient. The determination of efficacy or futility should be based on physiological outcome criteria, not quality of life criteria. As far as is reasonably possible, medical decision making should be based on the results of well-designed research trials that include sufficient numbers of cases to determine that CPR is of no benefit.[5]

Instituting and Discontinuing CPR

Determination of Death in the Prehospital Setting

For patients who suffer sudden cardiac arrest, the prompt initiation of CPR remains the standard of care except where rigor mortis, lividity, tissue decomposition, or obviously fatal trauma are present, since these are reliable criteria for the determination of death.[6] Unwitnessed deaths in the presence of serious, chronic, debilitating disease in the terminal stage of a fatal illness may be used as criteria for not instituting CPR. Successful resuscitation is rarely achieved for patients in traumatic cardiac arrest, except under specific clinical conditions.[7] Patients with valid No-CPR orders should not have CPR initiated in the prehospital setting.[8] Pronouncement of death requires direct communication with physician medical control unless local protocol dictates otherwise.

Brain death cannot be determined by prehospital personnel, and pupil status or other evidence of neurological activity should not be used for the determination of death in the prehospital setting.[9] Patients who are hypothermic should be aggressively resuscitated, even when long transport times are involved.

Discontinuing Basic Life Support

Rescuers who initiate BLS should continue until one of the following occurs:

1. Effective spontaneous circulation and ventilation have been restored.
2. Care is transferred to emergency medical responders or another trained person who continues BLS or initiates advanced life support.
3. Care is transferred to a physician who determines that resuscitation should be discontinued.
4. The rescuer is unable to continue resuscitation because of exhaustion, because environmental hazards endanger the rescuer, or because continued resuscitation would jeopardize the lives of others.
5. Reliable criteria for the determination of death are recognized.
6. A valid No-CPR order is presented to the rescuers.

There is ongoing debate about the efficacy of BLS beyond 30 minutes. Rescuers in remote environments and in some BLS ambulance services have long transport times before advanced life support can be instituted and are therefore unavailable for other calls. The risk of vehicular accidents during high-speed emergency transport must also be weighed against the likelihood of successful resuscitation after prolonged BLS resuscitative efforts. State or local EMS authorities should be encouraged to develop protocols for initiation and withdrawal of BLS in areas where advanced life support is not readily available, taking into account local circumstances, resources, and risk

to rescuers. Since defibrillators are now recommended as standard equipment on all ambulances, the absence of a "shockable" rhythm on the defibrillator/monitor after an adequate trial of CPR can be an additional criterion for withdrawing BLS.

Discontinuing Resuscitation in Hospitals

In hospital, CPR may be withheld or discontinued under the following circumstances:

1. Appropriate BLS and an adequate trial of advanced life support have been attempted but circulation has not been restored.
2. No physiological benefit from basic and advanced life support can be expected because the patient's vital functions are deteriorating despite maximum therapy. (For example, CPR would not restore circulation in a patient who suffered a cardiac arrest despite optimal treatment for progressive septic or cardiogenic shock.)
3. The patient's vital functions have begun to decline, the patient has a terminal condition, and it has been found in large, well-designed studies that patients with that condition do not survive when provided CPR. (For example, when CPR is attempted in patients with metastatic cancer, several large series have reported that no patients survived to hospital discharge.[10])

Often when family members are unwilling to accept an impending death, they do not consent to a No-CPR order. "Slow codes" or "sham codes" in which CPR is performed perfunctorily to appear that "everything was done" undermine the trust between healthcare providers and patients and should not be attempted. An initial attempt to test the responsiveness of the cardiovascular system should be made with the intent of successful resuscitation but promptly discontinued if shown to be of no benefit.[11]

Hospital Policy Regarding CPR

Hospitals are required by the Joint Commission on the Accreditation of Health Care Organizations to have written policies for No-CPR orders. These policies need to be reviewed periodically to reflect developments in medical technology, changes in guidelines for CPR, or changes in the law.

The policies should state that the attending physician should write No-CPR orders in the patient's chart. The rationale for the No-CPR order and other specific limits to care should be documented in the progress notes.[12] Oral No-CPR orders may be misunderstood and may place nurses and other healthcare workers in legal jeopardy. If the attending physician is not present, nurses may accept a No-CPR order over the telephone, with the understanding that the physician will sign the order promptly. No-CPR orders should be reviewed periodically, particularly if the patient's condition changes and especially before the patient undergoes anesthesia.[13]

A No-CPR order means only that CPR will not be initiated. It does not mean that other care should be limited. These orders should not lead to abandonment of patients or denial of appropriate medical and nursing care. They do not constitute "giving up." For many patients, interventions for diagnosis or treatment remain appropriate after a No-CPR order is written.

Hospitals are now required to have advisers, such as ethics committees, who can respond to requests for resolution of ethical questions. Ethics committees traditionally have been consultative and advisory and have been effective in organizing educational programs and developing hospital policies and guidelines regarding CPR.

CPR in Nursing Homes

Nursing homes should develop and implement institutional guidelines for providing CPR to their residents. Care plans for residents should be individualized; CPR may not be indicated for all residents. Guidelines for withholding or initiating CPR should be developed, based on clinical criteria and patient preferences.[14] All patients should be encouraged to clearly state whether they prefer resuscitation should the need arise.

Community Systems for Communicating No-CPR Orders

There is often confusion about whether the No-CPR order is transferred from the hospital to the prehospital setting. Prehospital settings include homes, nursing homes, and public places. There are problems with how to identify patients who have a No-CPR order.[15] The most commonly used method is a standard form that is available from health departments, EMS agencies, or physicians. Other methods are the use of a bracelet, an identification card, or a central registry. Healthcare providers and patients should be educated about appropriate documentation and authenticity of various No-CPR orders in their local system.

Sometimes a family may demand CPR despite the presence of a well-documented No-CPR order at the scene of an emergency. It may be appropriate in such cases to begin resuscitation and transport the patient to the hospital. Treatment can be withdrawn when the conflicts are resolved and the authenticity and legitimacy of the No-CPR order are validated.

Sometimes there is confusion about the difference between No-CPR orders and living wills. No-CPR orders are physician orders directed to healthcare personnel to withhold CPR specifically. Living wills are legal documents stating a patient's preference regarding medical care should he or she lose decision-making capacity.[16] Living wills require interpretation and formulation into a medical care plan. Confusion occurs when living wills (not No-CPR orders) are presented to ambulance personnel providing ECC. Because of their complexity, living wills often cannot be interpreted by ambulance personnel. Living wills often require an assessment of the patient's decision-making capacity, the presence of terminal illness, the identification of proxies, and the formulation of vague requests into specific treatment plans. Generally, prehospital emergency treatment should be initiated and the patient transported to the hospital for interpretation of the living will. State laws, local ordinances, or EMS policy regarding the applicability of living wills in the prehospital setting should be reviewed. Advance directives that include written notations by the patient or verbal requests by family members about what the patient would want generally do not meet the procedural requirements for withholding emergency medical care.

Legal Mandates

While the provision of medical care is guided by the standard of care determined by the medical profession, courts, legislative bodies, and regulatory agencies have increasingly influenced the practice of medicine. State courts have consistently upheld the patient's right to refuse medical care, and state living-will laws provide procedural guidelines for patients who wish to exercise this right to direct their medical care should they lose decision-making capacity. Living wills are statutorily defined documents providing very specific instructions by which people convey their requests in a fashion that is legally enforceable. The Federal Patient Self-determination Act requires various healthcare agencies to inform patients of their rights under state living-will laws.[17]

A number of states have enacted laws to protect from liability persons who render aid in an emergency. These laws are often termed "Good Samaritan" laws after the biblical story of the Samaritan that stopped to render aid to a stranger while other travelers passed him by (Luke

10:30-37). These laws are intended to encourage people to render aid in emergency situations.

Good Samaritan laws generally provide that persons who render aid at the scene of an emergency will not be liable for civil damages if they act in good faith, and not for remuneration, in rendering aid. The persons protected under these laws vary greatly from state to state. In some states the laws apply both to laypersons and healthcare and other professionals. In others they apply only to specific healthcare professionals, such as physicians, surgeons, or nurses, or to other professionals, such as firefighters, police officers, school personnel, or lifeguards. In still others the laws apply to laypersons or emergency service personnel ony if they have received certain training in emergency aid.

Some states allow protection only if the aid is provided at the scene of the emergency. In others it applies to aid provided at the hospital by persons who are not emergency department or hospital personnel.

Most Good Samaritan laws provide that the person rendering emergency aid must have provided it in good faith, must not have acted with the expectation of remuneration, must not have been the cause of the emergency, and must not have been willfully or wantonly negligent in providing the aid. Note, however, that a Good Samaritan law is unlikely to be useful in protecting against liability arising from teaching CPR.

Good Samaritan laws are a useful and important tool to encourage the administration of aid in emergency situations. However, as the above summary illustrates, *the laws vary significantly from state to state.* Therefore, healthcare and emergency personnel, as well as others who may need to use CPR, would be well advised to determine whether their state has a Good Samaritan law, and if so, what persons and activities are protected under their local law.

Conclusions

Ethical values should guide the initiation and withdrawal of CPR, with patient autonomy and the burden and benefit of treatment considered rather than the threat of legal liability. Patient autonomy is respected by providing appropriate informed consent, allowing surrogate decision-making, and honoring valid No-CPR orders. Important differences exist between No-CPR orders, living wills, and other advance directives. No-CPR orders are written by physicians to withhold CPR, whereas living wills and other advance directives require interpretation and development into a care plan. CPR should be promptly instituted for patients in cardiac arrest with these important exceptions: the presence of a No-CPR order, the presence of reliable criteria for the determination of death, or the reliable prediction of no benefit. EMS systems should provide mechanisms for the determination of death in all settings, criteria for instituting and discontinuing BLS, and criteria for honoring No-CPR orders. Education of physicians, EMS providers, other healthcare personnel, and the public is necessary regarding the appropriate indications for instituting and withdrawing CPR.[7]

References

1. Jonsen AR, Siegler M, Winslade WJ. *Clinical Ethics: A Practical Approach to Ethical Decisions in Clinical Medicine.* 2nd ed. New York, NY: Macmillan Publishing Co Inc; 1986:102-109.
2. The Hastings Center. *Guidelines on the Termination of Life-Sustaining Treatment and the Care of the Dying: A Report.* Briarcliff Manor, NY: The Hastings Center; 1987:16-34.
3. Evans AL, Brody BA. The do-not-resuscitate order in teaching hospitals. *JAMA.* 1985;253:2236-2239.
4. Guidelines for the appropriate use of do-not-resuscitate orders. Council on Ethical and Judicial Affairs, American Medical Association. *JAMA.* 1991;265:1868-1871.
5. Tomlinson T, Brody H. Futility and the ethics of resuscitation. *JAMA.* 1990;264:1276-1280.
6. Standards and guidelines for Cardiopulmonary Resuscitation and Emergency Cardiac Care. *JAMA.* 1986;255:298.
7. Cogbill TH, Moore EE, Millikan S, Cleveland HC. Rationale for selective application of emergency department thoracotomy in trauma. *J Trauma.* 1983;23:453-460.
8. Guidelines for 'do not resuscitate' orders in the prehospital setting. American College of Emergency Physicians. *Ann Emerg Med.* 1988;17:1106-1108.
9. Report of a special task force: guidelines for the determination of brain death in children. American Academy of Pediatrics Task Force on Brain Death in Children. *Pediatrics.* 1987;80:298-300.
10. Faber-Langendoen K. Resuscitation of patients with metastatic cancer: is a transient benefit still futile? *Arch Intern Med.* 1991;151:235-239.
11. Blackhall LJ. Must we always use CPR? *N Engl J Med.* 1987;317:1281-1285.
12. Lo B. Unanswered questions about DNR orders. *JAMA.* 1991;265:1874-1875.
13. Cohen CB, Cohen PJ. Do-not-resuscitate orders in the operating room. *N Engl J Med.* 1991;325:1879-1882.
14. Crimmins TJ. CPR policy in nursing homes. *Minn Med.* 1991;74:29,35.
15. Crimmins TJ. The need for a prehospital DNR system. *Prehosp Disaster Med.* 1990;5:47-48.
16. Orentlicher D. From the Office of the General Counsel: advance medical directives. *JAMA.* 1990;263:2365-2367.
17. Wolf SM, Boyle P, Callahan D, Fins JJ, Jennings B, Nelson JL, Barondess JA, Brock DW, Dresser R, Emanuel L, Johnson S, Lantos J, Mason DCR, Mezey M, Orentlicher D, Rouse F. Sources of concern about the Patient Self-Determination Act. *N Engl J Med.* 1991;325:1666-1671.

Safety during CPR training and in actual rescue situations in which CPR is provided has gained increased attention. This chapter discusses both these issues. Adherence to the following recommendations should minimize possible complications for instructors and students during CPR training and implementation. The recommendations for manikin decontamination and rescuer safety originally established in 1978 by the Centers for Disease Control and Prevention[1] were updated in 1983 and again in 1989 by the AHA, the American Red Cross, and the Centers for Disease Control and Prevention to minimize possible complications during CPR training and in actual emergencies.[2,3]

Disease Transmission During CPR Training

The 1980s saw a dramatic increase in inquiries about the possible role of CPR training manikins in transmitting diseases such as human immunodeficiency virus (HIV), hepatitis B virus (HBV), herpesviruses, and various upper and lower respiratory infections, such as influenza, infectious mononucleosis, and tuberculosis. To date, it is estimated that approximately 70 million people in the United States have had direct contact with manikins during CPR training courses. Use of these manikins has never been documented as being responsible for an outbreak or even an isolated case of bacterial, fungal, or viral disease.[3]

Under certain circumstances, however, manikin surfaces present a remote risk of disease transmission. Therefore, manikin surfaces should be cleaned and disinfected in a consistent way.

There are two important infection control considerations in CPR training. First, practice on manikins can result in contamination by the hands or oral fluids. If manikins are not cleaned properly between each use and after each class, these contaminants may be transmitted. Second, internal parts, such as the valve mechanisms and artificial lungs in manikin airways, invariably become contaminated during use. If not dismantled and cleaned or replaced after class, they may become sources of contamination for subsequent classes. There is no evidence, however, that manikin valve mechanisms produce aerosols even when air is forcibly expelled during chest compression. In addition, a number of manufacturers produce different types of training manikins. Since these manikins have unique features, instructors and training agencies rely heavily on the manufacturers' recommendations for use and maintenance, and these recommendations should be carefully followed.

The resistance levels of microorganisms such as HIV, HBV, and herpesvirus have not been fully characterized. Several intermediate-level disinfectants can be used to kill these microorganisms on manikins. However, those containing iodine may stain or otherwise damage plastic materials. Others containing formaldehyde or glutaraldehyde leave undesirable residues, odors, or toxicities that may affect students.[4-6]

Neither HBV or HIV is as resistant to disinfectant chemicals as previously thought.[2,4-8] Studies have shown that the primary retroviral agent that causes acquired immunodeficiency syndrome (AIDS), HIV, is comparatively delicate and is inactivated in less than 10 minutes at room temperature by a number of disinfectants, including those agents recommended for manikin cleaning.[9-12] It is emphasized that there is no evidence to date that HIV is transmitted by casual personal contact, indirect contact with inanimate surfaces, or the airborne route. CPR courses are conducted with detailed attention to reduce the risk of disease transmission by carefully following manikin manufacturers' guidelines. These adequately protect against transmission of HIV and HBV, as well as bacterial and fungal infections. These guidelines discuss sterilization of manikins and face masks and give practical pointers on how to minimize risk of disease transmission for the students participating. The guidelines are discussed in detail in the *Instructor's Manual for Basic Life Support*.

If these recommendations are consistently followed, students in each class should be able to use manikins whose cleanliness equals or exceeds that of properly cleaned eating utensils. The recommended disinfectant chemicals have been shown to be safe, effective, inexpensive, easily obtained, and well tolerated by students, instructors, and manikin surfaces when used properly. A more intense level of surface disinfection than that recommended is not warranted.

The risk of transmission of any infectious disease by manikin practice appears to be very low. Although millions of people worldwide have used training mani-kins in the last 25 years, there has never been a docu-mented case of transmission of bacterial, fungal, or viral disease by a CPR training manikin. Thus, in the absence of evidence of infectious disease transmis-sion, the lifesaving potential of CPR should continue to be vigorously emphasized and energetic efforts in sup-port of broad-scale CPR training should be continued.

Disease Transmission During Actual Performance of CPR

The vast majority of CPR performed in the United States is done by healthcare and public safety person-nel, many of whom assist in ventilation of respiratory and cardiac arrest victims about whom they have little or no medical information. A layperson is far less likely to perform CPR than healthcare providers. The layper-son who performs CPR, whether on an adult or pedia-tric victim, is most likely to do so in the home, where 70% to 80% of respiratory and cardiac arrests occur.[8] In these situations the lay rescuer commonly knows the victim and often knows about the victim's health. Researchers have found that there is little reluctance by lay rescuers to perform CPR on family members, even in the presence of vomitus or alcohol on the breath.[13]

The layperson who responds to an emergency in an unknown victim should be guided by individual moral and ethical values and knowledge of risks that may exist in various rescue situations. It is safest for the rescuer to assume that any emergency situation that involves exposure to certain body fluids has the poten-tial for disease transmission for both the rescuer and victim.

The greatest concern over the risk of disease trans-mission should be directed to persons who perform CPR frequently, such as healthcare providers, in both the hospital and prehospital settings. Providers of pre-hospital emergency health care include paramedics, emergency medical technicians, law enforcement per-sonnel, firefighters, lifeguards, and others whose jobs require them to perform first-response medical care. The risk of disease transmission from infected per-sons to providers of prehospital emergency health care should be no higher than that for those providing emergency care in the hospital if appropriate precau-tions are taken to prevent exposure to blood or other body fluids.

The probability that a rescuer (lay or professional) will become infected with HBV or HIV as a result of

performing CPR is minimal.[14] Although transmission of HBV and HIV between healthcare workers and patients as a result of blood exchange or penetration of the skin by blood-contaminated instruments has been documented,[15] transmission of HBV and HIV infection during mouth-to-mouth resuscitation has not been documented.[16]

Direct mouth-to-mouth resuscitation will likely result in exchange of saliva between the victim and rescuer. However, HBV-positive saliva has not been shown to be infectious even to oral mucous membranes, through contamination of shared musical instruments, or through HBV carriers.[16] In addition, saliva has not been implicated in the transmission of HIV after bites, percutaneous innoculation, or contamination of cuts and open wounds with saliva from HIV-infected patients.[17,18] The theoretical risk of infection is greater for salivary or aerosol transmission of herpes simplex, *Neisseria meningitidis,* and airborne diseases such as tuberculosis and other respiratory infections. Rare instances of herpes transmission during CPR have been reported.[19]

The emergence of multidrug-resistant tuberculo-sis[20,21] and the risk of tuberculosis to emergency work-ers[22] is a cause for concern. In most instances, transmission of tuberculosis requires prolonged close exposure as is likely to occur in households, but trans-mission to emergency workers can occur during resuscitative efforts by either the airborne route[22,23] or by direct contact. The magnitude of the risk is uncer-tain but probably low.

After performing mouth-to-mouth resuscitation on a person suspected of having tuberculosis, the care-giver should be evaluated for tuberculosis using stan-dard approaches based on the caregiver's baseline skin tests.[24] Caregivers with negative baseline skin tests should be retested 12 weeks later.

Preventive therapy should be considered for all per-sons with positive tests and should be started on all converters.[25] In areas where multidrug-resistant tuberculosis is common or after exposure to known multidrug-resistant tuberculosis, the choice of preven-tive therapeutic agent is uncertain, but some authori-ties suggest two or more agents.[26]

Performance of mouth-to-mouth resuscitation or invasive procedures can result in the exchange of blood between the victim and rescuer, especially in cases of trauma and if either has had breaks in the skin on or around the lips or soft tissues of the oral cavity mucosa. Thus, a theoretical risk of HBV and HIV transmission during mouth-to-mouth resuscitation exists.[27]

Because of the concern about disease transmission between victim and rescuer, rescuers with a duty to provide CPR should follow the precautions and guidelines established by the Centers for Disease Control[14] and the Occupational Safety and Health Administration. These guidelines include the use of barriers, such as latex gloves, and mechanical ventilation equipment, such as a bag-valve mask and other resuscitation masks with valves capable of diverting expired air from the rescuer. Rescuers who have an infection that may be transmitted by blood or saliva should not perform mouth-to-mouth resuscitation if circumstances allow other immediate or effective methods of ventilation.

Although the efficacy of barrier devices has not been documented conclusively, those with a duty to respond should be instructed during CPR training in the use of masks with one-way valves. Plastic mouth and nose covers with filtered openings are also available and may provide a degree of protection. Masks without one-way valves (including those with S-shaped devices) offer little, if any, protection and should not be considered for routine use. Since intubation obviates the need for mouth-to-mouth resuscitation and is more effective than the use of masks alone, early intubation is encouraged when equipment and trained professionals are available. Resuscitation equipment known or suspected to be contaminated with blood or other body fluids should be discarded or thoroughly cleaned and disinfected after each use.[28] Following these precautions and guidelines should further reduce the risk of disease transmission when providing CPR.

References

1. Centers for Disease Control. *Recommendations for Decontaminating Manikins Used in Cardiopulmonary Resuscitation: Hepatitis Surveillance, Report 42.* Atlanta, Ga: Centers for Disease Control; 1978:34-36.
2. Prevention of acquired immune deficiency syndrome (AIDS): report of inter-agency recommendations. *MMWR.* 1983;32:101-103.
3. Risk of infection during CPR training and rescue: supplemental guidelines. The Emergency Cardiac Care Committee of the American Heart Association. *JAMA.* 1989;262:2714-2715.
4. Bond WW, Petersen NJ, Favero MS. Viral hepatitis B: aspects of environmental control. *Health Lab Sci.* 1977;14:235-252.
5. Bond WW, Favero MS, Petersen NJ, Ebert JW. Inactivation of hepatitis B virus by intermediate-to-high-level disinfectant chemicals. *J Clin Microbiol.* 1983;18:535-538.
6. Favero MS, Bond WW. Sterilization, disinfection and antisepsis in the hospital. In: Balows A, Hausler WJ Jr, Hermann KL, Eisenberg HD, Shadomy HJ, eds. *Manual of Clinical Microbiology.* 5th ed. Washington, DC: American Society for Microbiology; 1991:183-200.
7. Acquired immune deficiency syndrome (AIDS): precautions for clinical and laboratory staffs. *MMWR.* 1982;31:577-580.
8. Standards and guidelines for cardiopulmonary resuscitation (CPR) and emergency cardiac care (ECC). *JAMA.* 1986; 255:2905-2984.
9. Resnick L, Veren K, Salahuddin SZ, Tondreau S, Markham PD. Stability and inactivation of HTLV-III/LAV under clinical and laboratory environments. *JAMA.* 1986;255:1887-1891.
10. Martin LS, McDougal JS, Loskoski SL. Disinfection and inactivation of the human T lymphotropic virus type III/ lymphadenopathy-associated virus. *J Infect Dis.* 1985;152:400-403.
11. McDougal JS, Cort SP, Kennedy MS, et al. Immunoassay for the detection and quantitation of infectious human retrovirus, lymphadenopathy-associated virus (LAV). *J Immunol Methods.* 1985;76:171-183.
12. Spire B, Dormont D, Barre-Sinoussi F, Montagnier L, Chermann JC. Inactivation of lymphadenopathy-associated virus by heat, gamma rays, and ultraviolet light. *Lancet.* 1985;1:188-189.
13. McCormack AP, Damon SK, Eisenberg MS. Disagreeable physical characteristics affecting bystander CPR. *Ann Emerg Med.* 1989;18:283-285.
14. Guidelines for prevention of transmission of human immunodeficiency virus and hepatitis B virus to health-care and public-safety workers. *MMWR.* 1989;38(suppl 6):1-37.
15. Marcus R. Surveillance of health care workers exposed to blood from patients infected with the human immunodeficiency virus. *N Engl J Med.* 1988;319:1118-1123.
16. Sande MA. Transmission of AIDS: the case against casual contagion. *N Engl J Med.* 1986;314:380-382.
17. Fox PC, Wolff A, Yeh CK, Atkinson JC, Baum BJ. Saliva inhibits HIV-1 infectivity. *J Am Dent Assoc.* 1988;116:635-637.
18. Friedland GH, Saltzman BR, Rogers MF, et al. Lack of transmission of HTLV-III/LAV infection to household contacts of patients with AIDS or AIDS-related complex with oral candidiasis. *N Engl J Med.* 1986;314:344-349.
19. Hendricks AA, Shapiro EP. Primary herpes simplex infection following mouth-to-mouth resuscitation. *JAMA.* 1980;243: 257-258.
20. Outbreak of multidrug-resistant tuberculosis—Texas, California, and Pennsylvania. *MMWR.* 1990;39:369-372.
21. Nosocomial transmission of multidrug-resistant tuberculosis among HIV–infected persons—Florida and New York, 1988-1991. *MMWR.* 1991;40:585-591.
22. Haley CE, McDonald RC, Rossi L, Jones WD Jr, Haley RW, Luby JP. Tuberculosis epidemic among hospital personnel. *Infect Control Hosp Epidemiol.* 1989;10:204-210.
23. Ehrenkranz NJ, Kicklighter JL. Tuberculosis outbreak in a general hospital: evidence for airborne spread of infection. *Ann Intern Med.* 1972;77:377-382.
24. Dooley SW Jr, Castro KG, Hutton MD, Mullan RJ, Polder JA, Snider DE Jr. Guidelines for preventing the transmission of tuberculosis in health-care settings, with special focus on HIV-related issues. *MMWR.* 1990;39:1-29.
25. The use of preventive therapy for tuberculosis infection in the United States: recommendations of the Advisory Committee for Elimination of Tuberculosis. *MMWR.* 1990;39:9-12.
26. Steinberg JL, Nardell EA, Kass EH. Antibiotic prophylaxis after exposure to antibiotic-resistant *Mycobacterium tuberculosis.* *Rev Infect Dis.* 1988;10:1208-1219.
27. Piazza M, Chirianni A, Picciotto L, Guadagnino V, Orlando R, Cataldo PT. Passionate kissing and microlesions of the oral mucosa: possible role in AIDS transmission. *JAMA.* 1989;261:244-245. Letter.
28. Recommendations for prevention of HIV transmission in healthcare settings. *MMWR.* 1987;36(suppl 2):1S-18S.

Automated External Defibrillation

Importance of Automated External Defibrillation

The AHA adds this chapter to the latest edition of the *Textbook of Basic Life Support for Healthcare Providers* because of greater awareness of the importance of early defibrillation and growing availability and use of automated external defibrillators (AEDs).[1-11] Every person trained in ACLS must be familiar with AEDs and know how to interact with emergency personnel equipped with these devices.

Defibrillation was once a skill reserved for emergency care providers trained in all aspects of ACLS, but it is now often performed by lesser-trained, BLS personnel.[5-7] The availability of AEDs has sparked this extension of defibrillation capability.[2] AEDs eliminate the need for training in rhythm recognition and make early defibrillation by minimally trained personnel practical and achievable.[1-11] AEDs were originally conceived as devices that would be used by emergency personnel and by family members and associates of people at high risk for sudden cardiac death.[12] Now the range of personnel who may be trained in the use of these devices is much broader.[13] Providers of ACLS, both in-hospital and prehospital, should be able to use AEDs and know the protocols for AED use because they may need to use these devices and because they will be called on with increasing frequency to interact with medical personnel or community members who also can use these devices.

Principle of Early Defibrillation

The principle of early defibrillation states that all BLS personnel must be trained to operate, equipped with, and permitted to operate a defibrillator if in their professional activities they are expected to respond to people in cardiac arrest. This concept has now achieved wide acceptance.[6,8,10,11,14-17] BLS personnel include all first-responding emergency personnel, whether in-hospital or out-of-hospital (eg, EMTs, non-EMT first-responders, firefighters, volunteer emergency personnel, physicians, nurses, and paramedics). Early defibrillation has become the standard of care for patients with either prehospital or in-hospital cardiac arrest,[18] except in sparsely populated and remote

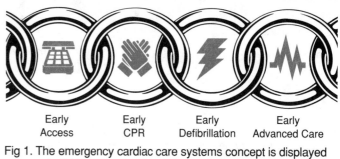

Fig 1. The emergency cardiac care systems concept is displayed schematically by the "chain of survival" metaphor.

settings where the frequency of cardiac arrest is low and rescuer response times are excessively long.[19-21]

ECC Systems Concept

The AHA has adopted and supported the ECC systems concept for years.[1,18] The phrase "chain of survival"[22] provides a useful metaphor for the elements of the ECC systems concept (Fig 1). The ECC systems concept summarizes the present understanding of the best approach to the treatment of persons with sudden cardiac death. The four links in this chain are early access to the EMS system, early CPR, early defibrillation, and early advanced cardiac care. Epidemiological and clinical research have established that effective ECC, whether prehospital or in-hospital, depends on strong links that are closely interconnected.[23-25] To achieve maximum effectiveness, each link must receive special attention. Through the education and training in its BLS program, the AHA strengthens the first two elements: early access and early CPR.[10,11] Through ACLS training, the fourth link, early advanced cardiac care, is established. Now, this educational material for automated defibrillation training strengthens the third component, early defibrillation. When the entire ECC system is brought together effectively, the potential for incremental improvement in survival from cardiac arrest is immense, as displayed in Fig 2.

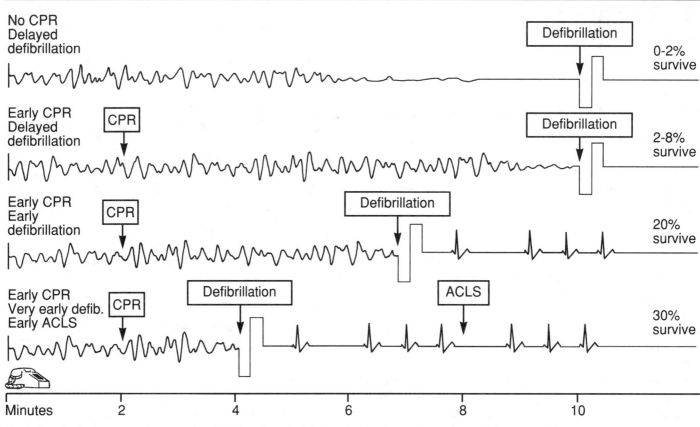

No CPR Delayed defibrillation — Defibrillation — 0-2% survive

Early CPR Delayed defibrillation — CPR — Defibrillation — 2-8% survive

Early CPR Early defibrillation — CPR — Defibrillation — 20% survive

Early CPR Very early defib. Early ACLS — CPR — Defibrillation — ACLS — 30% survive

Minutes   2   4   6   8   10

Fig 2. Survival rates are estimates of probability of survival to hospital discharge for patients with witnessed collapse and with ventricular fibrillation as initial rhythm. Estimates are based on a large number of published studies, which are collectively reviewed in References 26 and 27.

Rationale for Early Defibrillation

A simple rationale supports early defibrillation:

- The most frequent initial rhythm in sudden cardiac arrest is ventricular fibrillation.
- The most effective treatment for ventricular fibrillation is electrical defibrillation.
- The probability of successful defibrillation diminishes rapidly over time.
- Ventricular fibrillation tends to convert to asystole within a few minutes.

Many adult patients in ventricular fibrillation can survive neurologically intact even if defibrillation is performed as late as 6 to 10 minutes after the arrest.[23,28-31] CPR performed during this period of waiting for the defibrillator appears to extend the existence of ventricular fibrillation and to contribute to preservation of heart and brain function.[30-32] The use of basic CPR, however, cannot convert hearts in ventricular fibrillation to a normal rhythm.

The speed with which defibrillation is performed is a major determinant of the success of resuscitation attempts. Nearly all neurologically intact survivors,

who in some studies number more than 90%, were patients with a ventricular tachyarrhythmia that had been treated by emergency personnel.[23,28-31] It appears from studies in which Holter monitors were used that ventricular tachycardia is the initial rhythm disturbance[30] in approximately 85% of persons with sudden, out-of-hospital, nontraumatic cardiac arrest. Ventricular tachycardia, however, is frequently short lived and converts rapidly to ventricular fibrillation, from which the only hope for successful resuscitation lies in early defibrillation. Furthermore, the proportion of patients with ventricular fibrillation also declines with each passing minute as more and more of these patients deteriorate into asystole, from which successful resuscitation is extremely unlikely. The remaining nonventricular fibrillation patients have a low probability of survival with current resuscitation techniques. By 4 to 8 minutes after the attack, approximately 50% of patients are still in ventricular fibrillation.[10,11,24,25,28]

Survival rates from cardiac arrest can be remarkably high if the event is witnessed. For example, when people in supervised cardiac rehabilitation programs suffer a witnessed cardiac arrest, defibrillation is usually performed within minutes; in four studies of cardiac arrest in this setting, 90 of 101 victims (89%) were resuscitated.[33-36] This is the highest survival rate reported for a defined out-of-hospital population.

Improved survival rates of patients with cardiac arrest have been reported from communities that had no prehospital ACLS services but added early defibrillation programs. The most impressive results were reported from King County, Washington, where the survival rate of patients with ventricular fibrillation improved from 7% to 26%,[37] and from rural Iowa, where the survival rate for ventricular fibrillation rose from 3% to 19%.[38] More modest results have been observed in rural communities of southeastern Minnesota,[39] northeastern Minnesota,[40] and Wisconsin[41] (Table 1).

A major determinant in these studies was time. It is clear that the earlier defibrillation occurs, the better the prognosis. Emergency personnel have only a few min-

utes after the collapse of a person to reestablish a sustained perfusing rhythm (Fig 2). The use of CPR can sustain a patient for a short period of time but cannot directly restore an organized rhythm. Restoration of an adequate perfusing rhythm requires defibrillation and advanced cardiac care, which must be administered within a few minutes of the initial arrest. Table 2 compares the differences in survival observed in different types of EMS systems. These systems differ in how well they strengthen the chain of survival. Figure 3 displays the sequence of events that must occur to ensure a successful resuscitation from cardiac arrest. The use of AEDs increases the range of personnel who can use a defibrillator and thus shortens the time between collapse and defibrillation. This exciting prospect accounts for the addition of this material to the ACLS training curriculum.

Table 1. Effectiveness of Early Defibrillation Programs[17]

Location	Before Early Defibrillation		After Early Defibrillation		Odds Ratio for Improved Survival
King County, Wash	7		26	(10/38)	3.7
Iowa	3	(1/31)	19	(12/64)	6.3
Southeast Minnesota	4	(1/27)	17	(6/36)	4.3
Northeast Minnesota	2	(3/118)	10	(8/81)	5.0
Wisconsin	4	(32/893)	11	(33/304)	2.8

Values are percent surviving and, in parentheses, how many patients had ventricular fibrillation.

Table 2. Range of Survival Rate to Hospital Discharge for All Cardiac Arrests and Ventricular Fibrillation by System Type: Data From 29 Locations[26]

System Type	Survival: All Rhythms (%)	Weighted Average (%)	Survival: Ventricular Fibrillation (%)	Weighted Average (%)
EMT only	2-9	5	3-20	12
EMT-D	4-19	10	6-26	16
Paramedics	7-18	10	13-30	17
EMT/paramedic	4-26	17	23-33	26
EMT-D/paramedic	13-18	17	27-29	29

EMT indicates emergency medical technician; EMT-D, emergency medical technician-defibrillation.

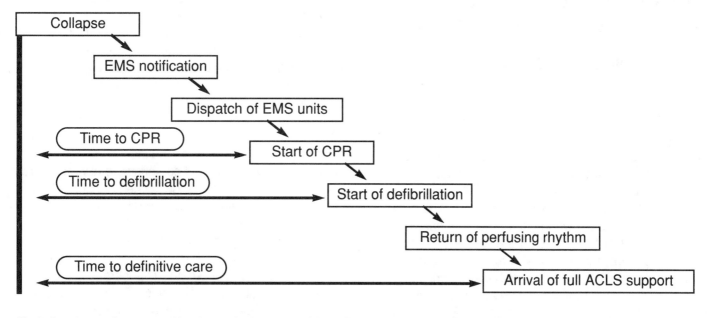

Fig 3. Sequence of events and key intervals that occur with cardiac arrest, based on Reference 27.

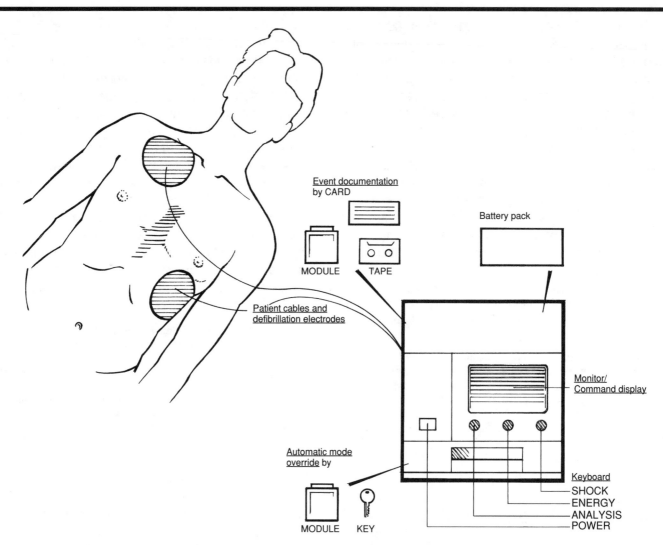

Fig 4. Schematic drawing of automated external defibrillator and its attachments to patient.

Overview of Automated External Defibrillators

Types of Automated External Defibrillators

The generic term "automated external defibrillators" refers to external defibrillators that incorporate a rhythm analysis system. Some devices are considered "fully" automated, whereas others are "semiautomated" or "shock-advisory" defibrillators.[42] All AEDs are attached to the patient by two adhesive pads and connecting cables,[43] as shown in Fig 4. These adhesive pads have two functions — to record the rhythm and to deliver the electric shock. A fully automated defibrillator requires only that the operator attach the defibrillatory pads and turn on the device. The device then analyzes the rhythm; if ventricular fibrillation (or ventricular tachy-cardia above a preset rate) is present, the device will charge its capacitors and deliver a shock.

Semiautomated or shock-advisory devices require additional operator steps, including pressing an "analyze" control to initiate rhythm analysis and pressing a "shock" control to deliver the shock. The shock control is pressed only when the device identifies ventricular fibrillation and "advises" the operator to press the shock control.

Fully automated defibrillators were developed with simple requirements for use by inexperienced operators. Primarily, this user group has comprised family members of high-risk patients and emergency personnel who are rarely called on to treat patients in cardiac arrest.

Shock-advisory AEDs may be safer because they never enter the analysis mode unless activated by the operator and they leave the final decision of whether to deliver the shock to the operator. This increase in safety is more theoretical than real because clinical experience suggests the devices are equally safe with or without a human operator to push the final shock button.[42]

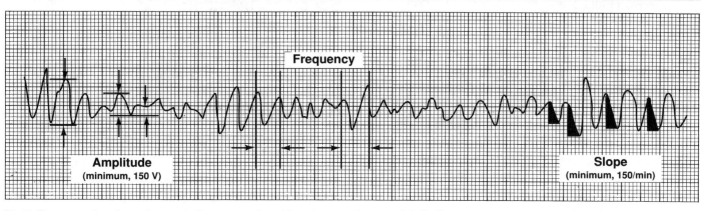

Fig 5. Features of surface electrocardiogram analyzed by automated external defibrillators.

Automated Analysis of Cardiac Rhythms

Unlike many other devices and approaches in emergency medicine, AEDs have been extensively tested, both in vitro against libraries of recorded cardiac rhythms[44] and clinically in numerous field trials.[39,45-52] The accuracy of the devices in rhythm analysis has been high. The rare errors noted with AEDs in field trials have been almost solely errors of omission where the device failed to recognize certain varieties of ventricular fibrillation or tachycardia.

The presently available AEDs are highly sophisticated, microprocessor-based devices that analyze multiple features of the surface ECG signal, including frequency, amplitude, and some integration of frequency and amplitude such as slope or wave morphology (Fig 5). A variety of filters check for QRS-like signals, radio transmission, or 60-cycle interference as well as for loose electrodes and poor electrode contact. Some devices are programmed to detect spontaneous patient movements, continued heartbeat and blood flow, or movement of the patient by others.

AEDs take multiple "looks" at the patient's rhythm, each look lasting a few seconds. If several of these analyses confirm the presence of a rhythm for which a shock is indicated and the other checks are consistent with a nonperfusing cardiac status, the fully automated defibrillator will charge and deliver a shock to the patient. The semiautomated devices will signal the operator that a shock is advised. It does this after charging the capacitors, which does not occur until appropriate ventricular fibrillation or tachycardia has been identified. Once the capacitors are charged, a shock is advised. The operator can then push a shock button, and the shock is delivered.

Inappropriate Shocks

Extensive clinical experience has revealed that AEDs are not misled by patient movements (eg, seizures and agonal respirations), by the patient being moved by others, or by artifactual signals.[45-52] Although the occurrence of inappropriate shocks in such circumstances has not been reported, AEDs should be placed in the analysis mode only when all movement, particularly the movement of patient transport, has ceased. The only major errors reported in clinical trials have been occasional failures to deliver shocks to rhythms that may benefit from electrical therapy, such as extremely fine or coarse ventricular fibrillation.

Ventricular Tachycardia

Although not designed to deliver synchronized shocks, all AEDs will shock monomorphic and polymorphic ventricular tachycardia if the rate is more than preset values. All rescuers who operate AEDs are trained to attach the device only to unconscious patients who are pulseless and apneic. With this approach, the operator serves as a second verification system to confirm that the patient has suffered a cardiac arrest. In an apneic, pulseless patient, electrical shocks are indicated whether the rhythm is supraventricular tachycardia, ventricular tachycardia, or ventricular fibrillation. There have been no reports of shocks delivered to conscious patients with perfusing ventricular or supraventricular dysrhythmias — a testament to good training and good patient-assessment skills of rescuers.

Interruption of CPR

Emergency personnel must not touch the patient while the AED analyzes the rhythm, charges the capacitors, and delivers the shocks. Chest compression and ventilation must cease while the device is operating; this permits accurate analysis of the cardiac rhythm and prevents accidental shocks to the rescuers. Movements induced by CPR can cause the AED to stop its analysis. The time between activating the rhythm analysis system, which is when CPR must stop, and the delivery of a shock averages 10 to 15 seconds.

This time without CPR that occurs with the use of AEDs is a recognized exception to the AHA guidelines, which recommend that CPR not be stopped for more than 5 seconds. With the use of AEDs, the negative effects of temporarily stopping CPR are outweighed by the positive effects of delivering an early defibrillatory shock. For patients in refractory ventricular fibrillation after the first shock, CPR may have to be interrupted for even longer periods of time to deliver the recommended three sequential shocks. Consequently, the standards for CPR and ECC accept a period of a maximum of 90 seconds for diagnosing ventricular fibrillation and delivering three shocks.[18,p2942]

Advantages and Disadvantages of Automated External Defibrillators

The major distinction between an automated and a conventional defibrillator is that a person must interpret the cardiac rhythm when a conventional defibrillator is used, but an electrical device interprets the rhythm when an AED is used.

Initial Training and Continuing Education

Conventional defibrillators require regular training and continuing education in rhythm recognition and device operation. The only psychomotor skills required by an AED user involve recognition of a cardiac arrest, proper attachment of the device, and adherence to the memorized treatment sequence. Learning to use and operate an AED is easier than learning to perform CPR.[53] Many of the advantages of AEDs stem from brief, convenient training sessions and continuing education.[54] In systems in which compensation must be provided for the initial training time and skills review classes, the use of AEDs offers considerable financial savings.[55] In systems in which the anticipated number of cardiac arrests is low, skills maintenance is a major concern.[19,20] AEDs offer considerable advantages in these situations because little continuing education is needed.

Speed of Operation

In clinical trials, emergency personnel using an AED deliver the first shock an average of 1 minute sooner than personnel using conventional defibrillators.[48,49]

Rhythm Detection

Two field studies have compared the rhythm detection ability of AEDs with that of emergency personnel.[48,49] Although AEDs have not achieved 100% accuracy in rhythm detection, they perform as well as EMTs who use conventional defibrillators.[48,49] The errors of AEDs have generally been limited to identification of very fine or very coarse ventricular fibrillation. Presently available AEDs have responded appropriately to perfusing rhythms and to cardiac arrest rhythms for which shocks are not indicated.

Remote Defibrillation Through Adhesive Pads

Another advantage of AEDs stems from the use of the adhesive defibrillatory pads attached to the patient by connecting cables.[56] This approach permits remote, "hands-off" defibrillation, which is a safer method from the operator's perspective, particularly in the close confines of aeromedical and ground transport vehicles. Adhesive defibrillatory pads may also offer consistently better paddle placement during a lengthy resuscitation attempt. Although some conventional defibrillators have adapters that permit operation through remote adhesive pads, they are not widely used. All AEDs, however, have adhesive monitor-defibrillatory pads. With adhesive pads, the operator cannot bear down with the heavy pressure that is required to use the paddles of conventional defibrillators. This pressure is recommended to lower the transthoracic resistance by improving contact between the electrodes and the skin, decreasing the intrathoracic volume, and bringing the paddles closer to each other. The adhesive pads offer comparable low impedance, however, due to their larger pad surface area.[57]

Rhythm Monitoring

In clinical settings that require frequent rhythm monitoring, the liquid crystal rhythm displays of some AEDs are less suitable than the bright cathode-ray displays of conventional defibrillators.

Use of Automated External Defibrillators During Resuscitation Attempts

Operational Steps

All AEDs can be operated by following four simple steps:

1. Turn on the power.
2. Attach the device.
3. Initiate analysis of the rhythm.
4. Deliver the shock, if indicated.

Different brands and models of AEDs have a variety of features and controls and may differ in characteristics such as paper strip recorders, rhythm display methods, energy levels, and messages to the operator. Operators can orient themselves best by understanding how each brand and model approaches the previously mentioned four steps.

Standard Operational Procedures

Compared with the Megacode resuscitation procedures for ACLS, resuscitation attempts in which AEDs are used are relatively simple because there are fewer therapeutic options when only automated defibrillation and basic CPR can be implemented.

Most response teams, including those in-hospital, in medical clinics, or out-of-hospital, consist of at least two persons. One team member operates the defibrillator, and one member begins BLS. No other activities, including setting up oxygen delivery systems, suction equipment, intravenous lines, or mechanical CPR devices, should take precedence over or delay rhythm analysis and defibrillation. Instead, these interventions should proceed simultaneously if possible. The rescuer responsible for defibrillation concentrates on operating the defibrillator, while other rescuers attend to airway management, ventilations, and chest compressions.

The rescuer places the AED close to the supine patient's left ear and performs the defibrillation protocols from the patient's left side. This position provides better access to the defibrillator controls and easier placement of the defibrillatory pads and allows the other rescuer room to perform CPR. However, this position may not be possible in all clinical settings.

Depending on the manufacturer, the AED is turned on by pressing a power switch or by lifting the monitor screen to the "up" position. This activates the voice-ECG tape recorder and permits environmental sounds and operator statements to be recorded along with the patient's cardiac rhythm.

The adhesive defibrillatory pads are opened quickly and attached first to the defibrillatory cables and then to the patient's chest. The pads are placed in a modified lead II position (upper-right sternal border and lower-left ribs over the apex of the heart). When the pads are attached, CPR should be stopped, and the analysis control should be pressed. All contact with the patient during analysis must be avoided. Assessment of the rhythms takes from 5 to 15 seconds, depending on the brand of the AED. If ventricular fibrillation is present, the device will announce that a shock is indicated by a written message, a visual alarm, or, often, a voice-synthesized statement.

The rescuer must always state loudly a "clear-the-patient" message, such as "I'm clear. You're clear. Everybody clear" or simply "Clear," before pressing the shock control. In most devices, pressing the analyze button initiates charging of the capacitors if a treatable rhythm is detected. The device shows that charging has started with a tone, a voice-synthesized message, or a light indicator. Shock delivery should produce a sudden contraction of the patient's musculature like that seen with the use of a conventional defibrillator. After the first shock is delivered, CPR is not restarted; instead, the analyze control is pressed immediately to start another rhythm analysis cycle. If ventricular fibrillation persists, the device will indicate this, and the "charging" and "shock indicated" sequence is repeated for the second and third shocks. The goal is to analyze quickly for any persisting rhythm treatable by electrical shocks (Fig 6).

Age and Weight Guidelines

Cardiac arrest in the pediatric age group is seldom caused by ventricular fibrillation. Defibrillation, therefore, is of minor importance in pediatric resuscitation and certainly should not take priority over airway clearance and maintenance. It is recommended that presently available AEDs not be used in pediatric cardiac arrest; they are not capable of the lower energy settings required for pediatric defibrillation. The recommended maximum energy level for defibrillatory shocks in children is 4 J/kg. AEDs now have a minimum energy level of 200 J, which is high for patients weighing less than 50 kg (110 lb). Most experienced EMS systems recommend the following approach, which is also recommended by the AHA: attach AEDs only to patients in cardiac arrest who are more than 12 years old or weigh more than 90 lb.

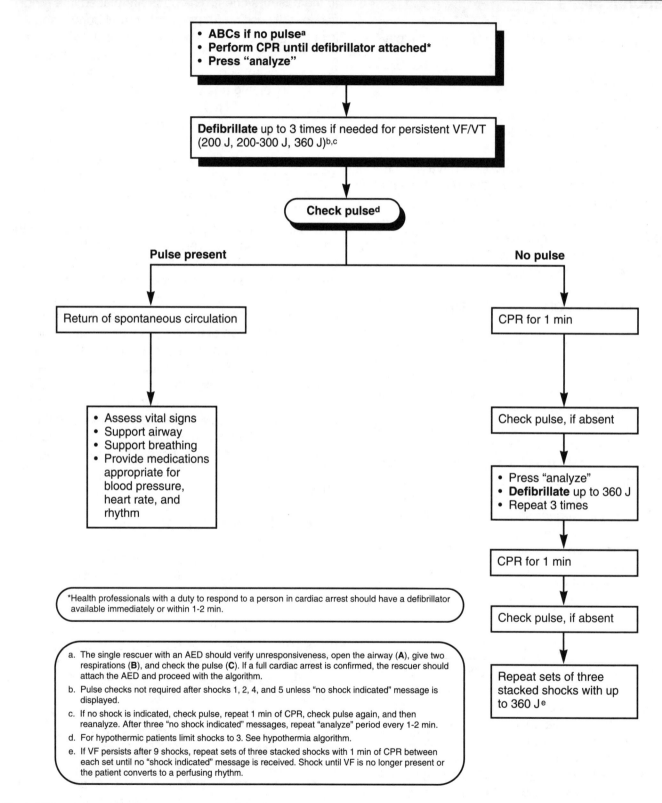

Automated External Defibrillation (AED) Treatment Algorithm
Emergency cardiac care pending arrival of ACLS personnel

- **ABCs if no pulse**[a]
- **Perform CPR until defibrillator attached***
- **Press "analyze"**

↓

Defibrillate up to 3 times if needed for persistent VF/VT (200 J, 200-300 J, 360 J)[b,c]

↓

Check pulse[d]

Pulse present / **No pulse**

Pulse present:

Return of spontaneous circulation

↓

- Assess vital signs
- Support airway
- Support breathing
- Provide medications appropriate for blood pressure, heart rate, and rhythm

No pulse:

CPR for 1 min

↓

Check pulse, if absent

↓

- Press "analyze"
- **Defibrillate** up to 360 J
- Repeat 3 times

↓

CPR for 1 min

↓

Check pulse, if absent

↓

Repeat sets of three stacked shocks with up to 360 J[e]

*Health professionals with a duty to respond to a person in cardiac arrest should have a defibrillator available immediately or within 1-2 min.

a. The single rescuer with an AED should verify unresponsiveness, open the airway (**A**), give two respirations (**B**), and check the pulse (**C**). If a full cardiac arrest is confirmed, the rescuer should attach the AED and proceed with the algorithm.

b. Pulse checks not required after shocks 1, 2, 4, and 5 unless "no shock indicated" message is displayed.

c. If no shock is indicated, check pulse, repeat 1 min of CPR, check pulse again, and then reanalyze. After three "no shock indicated" messages, repeat "analyze" period every 1-2 min.

d. For hypothermic patients limit shocks to 3. See hypothermia algorithm.

e. If VF persists after 9 shocks, repeat sets of three stacked shocks with 1 min of CPR between each set until no "shock indicated" message is received. Shock until VF is no longer present or the patient converts to a perfusing rhythm.

Fig 6. AED treatment algorithm.

Persistent Ventricular Fibrillation and No Available ACLS

The energy levels of the second and third shocks can range from 200 to 360 J. The guidelines for CPR and ECC recommend the use of 200 to 300 J for the second shock and an energy level "not to exceed 360 J" for a third shock if the first two shocks fail to defibrillate. Some AEDs are programmed to automatically increase the energy level to 360 J on the third shock. Others allow the operator to either remain at 200 J or increase the energy level for subsequent shocks. Neither approach has been established as superior. Some evidence suggests that lower energy shocks have a greater likelihood of leaving the patient in persistent ventricular fibrillation, whereas higher energy shocks may more frequently leave the patient in asystole.[58]

If no pulse returns after these three shocks, rescuers with AEDs but without immediate ACLS backup should not press the analysis button but should instead resume CPR for 60 seconds. They should then deliver additional rounds of three "stacked" defibrillatory shocks after the appropriate analysis period if ventricular fibrillation continues. Presently available AEDs will return to a sequence of 200-, 200-, and 360-J shocks at this point, although programmable modules allow a variety of protocols, depending on local practice. If the patient must be transported by the AED response team, then standing orders and guidelines will vary depending on local protocols.

AEDs can be left attached to the patient during transport in moving vehicles. However, AEDs should never be placed in the analyze mode in such circumstances because the movement of the transport vehicle can interfere with rhythm assessment. If a patient requires rhythm analysis and treatment during transport, then the vehicle must be brought to a complete stop. CPR should be administered during transport when indicated.

Recurrent Ventricular Fibrillation — Refibrillation With No Available ACLS

If the patient regains a perfusing rhythm after receiving shocks and at some later time refibrillates, the rescuer using an AED should restart the treatment sequence from the beginning.[53] Whenever the "no shock indicated" message is received, the rescuer should check for a pulse and, if there is none, resume CPR. Three "no shock indicated" messages indicate that there is a low probability that the rhythm present can be successfully shocked. Therefore, the rhythm

analysis time periods should be repeated only at 1- to 3-minute intervals.

Single Rescuer With an Automated External Defibrillator

In some situations, a single rescuer equipped with or with immediate access to an AED may have to respond to a person in cardiac arrest. Traditional BLS guidelines recommended that whenever the rescuer is alone, "CPR should be performed for about 1 minute and then help should be summoned."[18,p2919] The purpose of this 1 minute of CPR was to provide circulation of oxygenated blood before efforts to activate the EMS system. Activation of the EMS system, in turn, aims to get a defibrillator to the patient as fast as possible. Because defibrillation, in the form of the AED, is already available, the minute of CPR and the immediate activation of the EMS system become of less importance. The need for rapid identification and defibrillation of shockable rhythms dictates attachment of the AED and analysis of the rhythm before 1 minute of CPR. A full cardiac arrest with an unobstructed airway must be confirmed. The prescribed period of CPR by the lone rescuer, however, can be omitted. Consequently, the rescue sequence becomes verify unresponsiveness, open the airway, give two respirations, and check the pulse. If no pulse, attach the AED and proceed with the algorithm for ventricular fibrillation and pulseless ventricular tachycardia (Fig 6). Activation of the EMS system should occur whenever the "no shock indicated" message is displayed or when someone else arrives on the scene.

No Pulse Checks Between Shocks

The ACLS Subcommittee Task Force on Early Defibrillation recommended that there be no pulse check between the stacked shocks, that is, after shocks 1, 2, 4, and 5. The conventional ACLS ventricular fibrillation protocols require a pulse check after these shocks because the leads may have become dislodged, an artifact may be producing "false" ventricular fibrillation, or an unrecognized perfusing rhythm may have returned. These sources of error do not occur with the use of AEDs. They have sensors to detect loose electrodes, artifactual rhythms, and regular rhythms associated with return of palpable pulse. Mandating a pulse check between shocks for AEDs will delay rapid identification of persistent ventricular fibrillation, interfere with the assessment capabilities of the devices, and increase the possibility of operator errors.

Summary of Standard Operational Procedures

The rescuer using an AED in the absence of ACLS can memorize an easy treatment sequence:

1. Attach AEDs only to people in apparent cardiac arrest.
2. Always shock in sets of three.
3. Every time the chest is touched after the first assessment, it should be to perform CPR for 1 minute.
4. Continue to shock until the "no shock" indicated message is received unless the patient is being transported to a close hospital.

Coordination of ACLS-Trained Provider With Personnel Using Automated External Defibrillators

With the increasing availability of AEDs, ACLS-trained emergency personnel will interact more frequently with AED-trained personnel. The following guidelines are suggested for this interface between ACLS personnel and personnel using AEDs.

1. ACLS-trained (and authorized) providers always have authority over the scene.
2. On arrival, ACLS-trained providers should ask for a quick report from the automated defibrillation providers and direct them to proceed with their protocols. This is particularly applicable when ACLS-trained providers are unfamiliar with the operation of the AED.
3. ACLS-trained providers should use the AED for additional shocks and rhythm monitoring. They can direct the providers to operate the AED. To save time, avoid disorganization, and allow a coordinated transfer of care, ACLS providers should not remove the AED and attach a separate conventional defibrillator, unless the AED in use lacks a rhythm display screen. Most AEDs have the capacity for "manual override" by ACLS-trained providers, should that be necessary. The method and ease for manual override will vary among models.
4. ACLS-trained providers should consider the shocks delivered by the AED operators as part of their ACLS protocols. For example, if the patient remains in ventricular fibrillation after three shocks by the AED, then the ACLS personnel should enter the ACLS ventricular fibrillation treat-

ment sequence at the point at which the first three shocks have been delivered. Consequently, ACLS providers should move immediately to establish intravenous line access, administer epinephrine, and perform endotracheal intubation.
5. In most circumstances, the AED should be removed and a conventional defibrillator attached only when the patient has regained a spontaneous rhythm or is ready for transport to another location or when the ACLS provider has reason to believe the AED is malfunctioning. Some models of AEDs lack a rhythm display monitor; thus, ACLS personnel will want to attach a conventional defibrillator when clinically convenient.

Postresuscitation Care

Once an automated external defibrillation provider team completes its protocol, several things could happen. Patients could display a maximal response to resuscitation and be awake, responsive, and breathing spontaneously; a palpable pulse may be restored with a variety of hemodynamic profiles and thus a variety of neurological and respiratory responses; cardiac arrest may persist without a rhythm that will respond to shocks; or a pulseless ventricular tachycardia or fibrillation may remain. In each event, patient care remains paramount. If the patient regains a pulse, the resuscitation team will continue to provide supportive care with one or a combination of the following.

- Proper airway control and ventilatory management
- Supplemental oxygen, if available
- Appropriate airway clearance if vomiting occurs
- Continued monitoring of vital signs
- Physical stabilization and transport
- Continued support while awaiting the arrival of the ACLS team

Training

Sources of Information

AHA training materials on AEDs are provided in the *Instructor's Manual for Basic Life Support* .

The instructor's manual includes a detailed instructor's curriculum and instructor's guidelines for a separate provider's course on AEDs. The AHA does not intend to approve, control, or directly supervise such courses because EMS agencies of most states already provide these functions. Instead, this material is intended to provide a standardized, national curriculum and course content that can be adapted for local use. It is hoped that the AHA-approved algorithms and recommendations for the proper use of AEDs will lead to greater national uniformity in the use of these devices.

General Points About Training

Because of the intrinsic simplicity of AEDs, a markedly expanded range of individuals can now be trained to provide early defibrillation. Individuals who may want training in the use of AEDs include general hospital floor nurses, general office nurses, oral surgeons, dentists, physician assistants, nurse practitioners, security and law enforcement personnel, ship and airplane crews, supervisory personnel at senior citizen centers and exercise facilities, and the entire range of professional prehospital providers, including first-responders, firefighters, and EMTs. In addition, physicians who are not involved in daily emergency care but nevertheless perceive themselves at risk of encountering a patient in cardiac arrest may be interested in learning to use AEDs.

Maintenance of Skills

Survey results and experience in rural communities have demonstrated that depending on the rate of cardiac arrest in a community, an emergency responder may go several years without treating a patient in cardiac arrest.[19,21] Therefore, every program director must determine how to ensure correct performance when such an event occurs. Principles of adult education suggest that frequent practice of a psychomotor skill such as operating an AED in a simulated cardiac arrest offers the best skill maintenance.

Practice Frequency

The frequency and content of these practice sessions have been established by several successful programs.[6,19,37] At the present time, most systems permit a maximum of 90 days between practice drills and have found this to be satisfactory. Note that this is a maximum interval between drills. Many emergency personnel and systems drill as often as once a month. The most successful long-term skill maintenance occurs when individual rescuers voluntarily take a few minutes to perform a quick check of the equipment on a frequent and regular basis. This check includes a visual inspection of the defibrillator components and controls and a mental review of the steps to be followed and the controls to be operated in the event of a cardiac arrest.

Session Content

The practice sessions can be as elaborate as interest and time allow and can include more advanced discussions of ECC. The following is recommended as a minimum content of a 30- to 60-minute practice session that should occur at least once every 90 days.

- Performance review of recent patients
- Review of equipment operation and maintenance
- Review of standing orders
- Discussion of treatment possibilities
- Scenario practice of field protocols with a training manikin, a defibrillator, and a rhythm simulator. This practice should simulate actual cardiac arrests and include entrance to the scene, two-person response teams, ongoing CPR, a variety of initial rhythms, and a variety of postshock responses
- An objective skills test, with a skills checklist (see the instructor's manual)

Medical Control

In emergencies, critical medical procedures must be performed by the first trained personnel who respond. Within the constraints of state law, health providers can perform some medical procedures in emergencies but only with the medical authorization of a physician. The authorizing physician assumes medical control and takes legal responsibility for the performance of the emergency care providers. The authorizing physician issues standing orders, which are in effect direct orders to perform specified tasks for a patient. The emergency rescuer must always operate under the authority of the medical license of the medical director and the enabling administrative codes of the state.

Successful Completion of Course

The AHA does **not** provide medical control for interventions taught in BLS or ACLS classes. "Successful completion" of an AHA course, including any automated external defibrillation provider's course that follows AHA recommendations, means only that a certain level of cognitive and performance standards has been met. Successful completion does not warrant performance, nor does it qualify or authorize a person to perform any procedure on a patient. Licensure and certification is a function of the appropriate state legislative or local health or EMS authority. Such licensure and certification may or may not be related to successful completion of a course following ACLS guidelines. The primary objectives of any automated defibrillation provider's course that follows AHA recommendations are educational.

Case-by-Case Review

Every event in which an AED is used (or could have been used) must be reviewed by the medical director or designated representative. This means that every incident in which CPR is performed must have a medical review to establish whether the patient was treated in accordance with professional standards and local standing orders. In each review, whether ventricular fibrillation and other rhythms were treated appropriately with shocks and with BLS must be considered. Other dimensions of performance that can be evaluated include command of the scene, safety, efficiency, speed, professionalism, ability to troubleshoot, completeness of patient care, and interactions with other professionals and bystanders.[59]

Methods of Case-by-Case Review

The three ways in which the case-by-case review is performed are by a written report, by review of the recordings made by the voice-ECG tape recorders attached to AEDs, and by solid-state memory modules and magnetic tape recordings that store information about each use of the device. The latter two methods are innovative approaches to event documentation, recordkeeping, and data management that have been recently developed and incorporated into AEDs.[59] Case reviews that use all three approaches appear to offer the most complete information. Particular requirements or constraints in some systems, however, may dictate various combinations of these approaches rather than all three. Future innovations in event documentation, such as digital voice recordings, annotated rhythm strips, and other microprocessor-based approaches, offer even more options.

Quality Assurance

Quality assurance refers to both the microperformance, that is, the performance of personnel involved in the treatment of individual patients, and the macroperformance, that is, the overall effectiveness of a system that uses AEDs. Quality assurance requires establishment of a system's performance goals, a review to determine whether those goals are being met, and feedback to move the system closer to unmet goals.[54] Review of the treatment of an individual patient in cardiac arrest can lead to identification of a problem in a system's training program.

Organized collection and review of patient data can identify systemwide problems and allow assessment of each link in the chain of survival for the adult victim of sudden cardiac death. Figure 7 presents the recommended minimum data that a system should obtain on cardiac arrest patients. Adult victims of witnessed cardiac arrest of presumed heart etiology and caused by ventricular fibrillation appear to be the best group on which to focus. The lower-than-expected hospital discharge rates of this group may be explained by long ambulance response times, delayed EMS activation, infrequent witnessed arrests, rare bystander CPR, or slow on-scene performance. Each of these problems can be addressed with a specific programwide effort. Continued systematic and uniform data collection will determine whether the new efforts succeed.

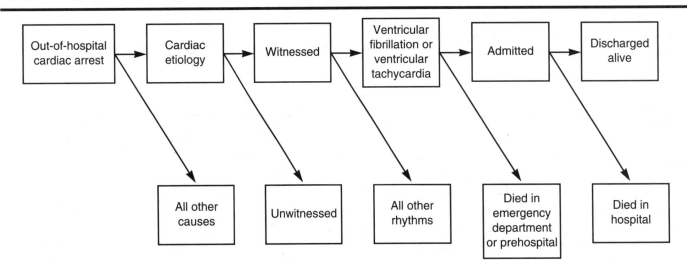

Fig 7. Recommended uniform data reporting approach for out-of-hospital cardiac arrest, based on data from Reference 27.

References

1. Atkins JM. Emergency medical service systems in acute cardiac care: state of the art. *Circulation.* 1986;74(suppl IV): IV-4-IV-8.

2. Cummins RO, Eisenberg MS, Stults KR. Automatic external defibrillators: clinical issues for cardiology. *Circulation.* 1986;73:381-385.

3. White RD. EMT-defibrillation: time for controlled implementation of effective treatment. *American Heart Association Emergency Cardiac Care National Faculty Newsletter.* 1986;8:1-3.

4. Atkins JM, Murphy D, Allison EJ Jr, Graves JR. Toward earlier defibrillation. *Emerg Med Serv.* 1986;11:70.

5. Eisenberg MS, Cummins RO. Defibrillation performed by the emergency medical technician. *Circulation.* 1986;74(suppl IV):IV-9-IV-12.

6. Cummins RO. EMT defibrillation: national guidelines for implementation. *Am J Emerg Med.* 1987;5:254-257.

7. Ruskin JN. Automatic external defibrillators and sudden cardiac death (editorial). *N Engl J Med.* 1988;319:713-715.

8. Cummins RO, Eisenberg MS. EMT defibrillation: a proven concept. *American Heart Association Emergency Cardiac Care National Faculty Newsletter.* 1984;1:1-3.

9. Cummins RO, Eisenberg MS, Moore JE, Hearne TR, Andresen E, Wendt R, Litwin PE, Graves JR, Hallstrom AP, Pierce J. Automatic external defibrillators: clinical, training, psychological, and public health issues. *Ann Emerg Med.* 1985;14:755-760.

10. Newman MM. National EMT-D study. *J Emerg Med Serv.* 1986;11:70-72.

11. Newman MM. The survival advantage: early defibrillation programs in the fire service. *J Emerg Med Serv.* 1987;12:40-46.

12. Cummins RO, Eisenberg MS, Bergner L, Hallstrom AP, Hearne T, Murray JA. Automatic external defibrillation: evaluations of its role in the home and in emergency medical services. *Ann Emerg Med.* 1984;13:798-801.

13. Jacobs L. Medical, legal and social implications of automatic external defibrillators (editorial). *Ann Emerg Med.* 1986;15: 863-864.

14. ACT (Advanced Coronary Treatment Foundation). EMT defibrillation — ACT Foundation issues policy statement. *J Emerg Med Serv.* 1983;8:37.

15. American College of Emergency Physicians EMS Committee. Prehospital defibrillation by basic-level emergency medical technicians. *Ann Emerg Med.* 1984;13:974.

16. Paris PM. EMT-defibrillation: a recipe for saving lives. *Am J Emerg Med.* 1988;6:282-287.

17. Cummins RO. From concept to standard-of-care? review of the clinical experience with automated external defibrillators. *Ann Emerg Med.* 1989;18:1269-1275.

18. American Heart Association. Standards and guidelines for cardiopulmonary resuscitation (CPR) and emergency cardiac care (ECC). *JAMA.* 1986;255:2905-2984.

19. Stults KR, Brown DD. Special considerations for defibrillation performed by emergency medical technicians in small communities. *Circulation.* 1986;74(suppl IV):IV-13-IV-17.

20. Ornato JP, McNeill SE, Craren EJ, Nelson NM. Limitations on effectiveness of rapid defibrillation by emergency medical technicians in a rural setting. *Ann Emerg Med.* 1984;13: 1096-1099.

21. Cummins RO, Eisenberg MS, Graves JR, Damon SK. EMT-defibrillation: is it right for you? *Emerg Med Serv.* 1985;10: 60-64.

22. Newman MM. The Chain of Survival concept takes hold. *J Emerg Med Serv.* 1989;14:11-13.

23. Eisenberg MS, Bergner L, Hallstrom AP. Paramedic programs and out-of-hospital cardiac arrest: I. factors associated with successful resuscitation. *Am J Public Health.* 1979;69:31-38.

24. Eisenberg MS, Bergner L, Hallstrom AP. Paramedic programs and out-of-hospital cardiac arrest: II. impact on community mortality. *Am J Public Health.* 1979;69:39-42.

25. Eisenberg MS, Copass MK, Hallstrom AP, Cobb LA, Bergner L. Management of out-of-hospital cardiac arrest: failure of basic emergency medical technician services. *JAMA.* 1980; 2243:1049-1051.

26. Eisenberg MS, Horwood BT, Cummins RO, Reynolds-Haertle R, Hearne TR. Cardiac arrest and resuscitation: a tale of 29 cities. *Ann Emerg Med.* 1990;19:179-186.

27. Eisenberg MS, Cummins RO, Damon S, Larsen MP, Hearne TR. Survival rates from out-of-hospital cardiac arrest: recommendations for uniform definitions and data to report. *Ann Emerg Med.* 1990;19:1249-1259.

28. Eisenberg MS, Hallstrom AP, Copass MK, Bergner L, Short F, Pierce J. Treatment of ventricular fibrillation: emergency medical technician defibrillation and paramedic services. *JAMA.* 1984;251:1723-1726.

29. Weaver WD, Copass MK, Bufi D, Ray R, Hallstrom AP, Cobb LA. Improved neurologic recovery and survival after early defibrillation. *Circulation.* 1984;69:943-948.

30. Cobb LA, Werner JA, Trobaugh GB. Sudden cardiac death: I. a decade's experience with out-of-hospital resuscitation. *Mod Concepts Cardiovasc Dis.* 1980;49:31-36.

31. Cobb LA, Hallstrom AP. Community-based cardiopulmonary resuscitation: what have we learned? *Ann NY Acad Sci.* 1982;382:330-342.

32. Bayes de Luna A, Coumel P, Leclercq JF. Ambulatory sudden cardiac death: mechanisms of production of fatal arrhythmia on the basis of data from 157 cases. *Am Heart J.* 1989;117: 151-159.

33. Fletcher GF, Cantwell JD. Ventricular fibrillation in a medically supervised cardiac exercise program: clinical, angiographic, and surgical correlations. *JAMA.* 1977;238:2627-2629.

34. Haskell WL. Cardiovascular complications during exercise training of cardiac patients. *Circulation.* 1978;57:920-924.

35. Hossack KF, Hartwig R. Cardiac arrest associates with supervised cardiac rehabilitation. *J Cardiac Rehab.* 1982;2:402-408.

36. Van Camp SP, Peterson RA. Cardiovascular complications of outpatient cardiac rehabilitation programs. *JAMA.* 1986;256: 1160-1163.

37. Eisenberg MS, Copass MK, Hallstrom AP, Blake B, Bergner L, Short FA, Cobb LA. Treatment of out-of-hospital cardiac arrests with rapid defibrillation by emergency medical technicians. *N Engl J Med.* 1980;302:1379-1383.

38. Stults KR, Brown DD, Schug VL, Bean JA. Prehospital defibrillation performed by emergency medical technicians in rural communities. *N Engl J Med.* 1984;310:219-223.

39. Vukov LF, White RD, Bachman JW, O'Brien PC. New perspectives on rural EMT defibrillation. *Ann Emerg Med.* 1988;17:318-321.

40. Bachman JW, McDonald GS, O'Brien PC. A study of out-of-hospital cardiac arrests in northeastern Minnesota. *JAMA.* 1986;256:477-483.

41. Olson DW, Larochelle J, Fark D, Aprahamian C, Aufderheide TP, Mateer JR, Hargarten KM, Stueven HA. EMT-defibrillation: the Wisconsin experience. *Ann Emerg Med.* 1989;18: 806-811.

42. Stults KR, Cummins RO. Fully automatic vs shock advisory defibrillators — what are the issues? *J Emerg Med Serv.* 1987;12:71-73.

43. Stults KR, Brown DD, Cooley F, Kerber RE. Self-adhesive monitor defibrillation pads improve prehospital defibrillation success. *Ann Emerg Med.* 1987;16:872-877.

44. Cummins RO, Stults KR, Haggar B, Kerber RE, Schaeffer S, Brown DD. A new rhythm library for testing automatic external defibrillators: performance of three devices. *J Am Coll Cardiol.* 1988;11:597-602.

45. Diack AW, Welborn WS, Rullman RG, Walter CW, Wayne MA. An automatic cardiac resuscitator for emergency treatment of cardiac arrest. *Med Instrum.* 1979;13:78-83.

46. Jaggarao NS, Heber M, Grainger R, Vincent R, Chamberlain DA. Use of an automated external defibrillator-pacemaker by ambulance staff. *Lancet.* 1982;2:73-75.

47. Cummins RO, Eisenberg M, Bergner L, Murray JA. Sensitivity, accuracy and safety of an automatic external defibrillator: report of a field evaluation. *Lancet.* 1984;2:318-320.

48. Stults KR, Brown DD, Kerber RE. Efficacy of an automated external defibrillator in the management of out-of-hospital cardiac arrest: validation of the diagnostic algorithm and initial clinical experience in a rural environment. *Circulation.* 1986; 73:701-709.

49. Cummins RO, Eisenberg MS, Litwin PE, Graves JR, Hearne TR, Hallstrom AP. Automatic external defibrillators used by emergency medical technicians: a controlled clinical trial. *JAMA.* 1987;257:1605-1610.

50. Gray AJ, Redmond AD, Martin MA. Use of the automatic external defibrillator-pacemaker by ambulance personnel: the Stockport experience. *Br Med J.* 1987;294:1133-1135.

51. Weaver WD, Hill D, Fahrenbruch CE, Copass MK, Martin JS, Cobb LA, Hallstom AP. Use of the automatic external defibrillator in the management of out-of-hospital cardiac arrest. *N Engl J Med.* 1988;319:661-666.

52. Jakobsson J, Nyquist O, Rehnqvist N. Effects of early defibrillation of out-of-hospital cardiac arrest patients by ambulance personnel. *Eur Heart J.* 1987;8:1189-1194.

53. Stults KR, Brown DD. Refibrillation managed by EMT-D's: incidence and outcome without paramedic backup. *Am J Emerg Med.* 1986;4:491-495.

54. Bradley K, Sokolow AE, Wright KJ, McCullough WJ. A comparison of an innovative four-hour EMT-D course with a 'standard' ten-hour course. *Ann Emerg Med.* 1988;17:613-619.

55. Ornato JP, Craren EJ, Gonzalez ER, Garnett AR, McClung BK, Newman MM. Cost-effectiveness of defibrillation by emergency medical technicians. *Am J Emerg Med.* 1988; 6:108-112.

56. Kerber RE, Martins JB, Kelly KJ, Ferguson DW, Kouba C, Jensen SR, Newman B, Parke JD, Kieso R, Melton J. Self-adhesive preapplied electrode pads for defibrillation and cardioversion. *J Am Coll Cardiol.* 1984;3:815-820.

57. Wilson RF, Sirna S, White CW, Kerber RE. Defibrillation of high risk patients during coronary angiography using self-adhesive preapplied electrode pads. *Am J Cardiol.* 1987;60: 380-382.

58. Weaver WD, Cobb LA, Copass MK, Hallstrom AP. Ventricular defibrillation — a comparative trial using 185-J and 320-J shocks. *N Engl J Med.* 1982;307:1101-1106.

59. Cummins RO, Austin D Jr, Graves JR, Hambly C. An innovative approach to medical control: semiautomatic defibrillators with solid-state memory for recording cardiac arrest events. *Ann Emerg Med.* 1988;17:818-824.